Additional Praise for *Being Fulfilled...*

"Jeff delivers some straightforward, no-nonsense, use-now strategies for *Being Fulfilled.* If you are serious about your results, study and practice what Jeff teaches… it will be invaluable to your sustained success."
-Dr. Denis Waitley, Author, *The Seeds of Greatness*

"Over the years, authors have sent me quite a number of books to review, and it has been hard, if not impossible, to write much about another book that covers the same old tired topics. Jeffrey's book, however, caught me off guard. It represents a fresh, clean look at personal fulfillment. Seen through his eyes as a personal coach and fitness professional of the highest caliber, he talks about building a life worth striving for, using easy exercises and relevant examples that everyone will be able to relate to.

It's a great book for anyone who has read, and is tired of, all the 'feel good' books that leave you wondering what you can do next. You'll find it at first a simple read, and then you'll realize that this book is worth reading again and again. Jeffrey makes sense, and this will be the first of many books and insights to come from his experience and wisdom."

-Thomas Plummer, Founder, National Fitness Business Alliance

"In a field full of highly energetic and enthusiastic people, Jeff has found a way to rise above them all. He has the ability to see what is unique and special about each individual he works with. Most importantly, he empowers his clients to use those traits to create positive growth. If you have the opportunity to work with Jeff, I have no doubt that you will find it to be inspiring."

-Beth Marie Oliver, Fitness Manager, Nike Sports Centers

"Being Fulfilled is a must-read for everyone attempting to juggle the fast pace of today's world. Jeffrey's approach and wisdom belies his age. He articulates the thought process and steps necessary to set priorities and succeed in the three critical areas of your life."

-Rich Boggs, CEO The Step Company

"Being Fulfilled provides a concrete and achievable direction for living a fulfilled life. Jeff's message is clear and simple: focus on a few vital responsibilities rather than on many trivial ones. This will produce real results… and true fulfillment in your life!"

-Harvey Diamond, Author, *Fit for Life*

"So many people strive for financial success and no matter how much money they make, end up broke inside because most neglect their relationships and above all their health. Jeff does an incredible job of showing you how to truly create a fulfilling life with fresh ideas and exciting strategies that work!"

-Jim Britt, Author, *Do This. Get Rich!*

"It becomes easy to put one's personal health and well being on the back burner while striving for business success. Jeff clearly and convincingly reveals how success and peak performance are directly related to our health."

-Bruce D Schneider, M.C.C., Author of *Energy Leadership: Transforming Your Workplace and Your Life from the Core*, and founder of iPEC Coaching

"I have had the absolute privilege of coaching and mentoring Jeffrey St.Laurent. He delivers a very unique message about the connection between mind, body and prosperity you deserve to receive. Jeff has overcome his own obstacles to be able to connect with you so you can become the person you deserve to be!"

-Jeffrey Combs, President, Golden Mastermind Seminars, inc., *www.GoldenMastermind.com*

"If you have ever said, "I'll start on Monday" or procrastinated about something for too long, Jeff will unequivocally inspire you to begin now! Jeff openly uncovers the true reality of what it takes to feel completely fulfilled in life… and best of all… how specifically to achieve it."

-Ron White, World memory expert, *www.RonWhiteTraining.com*

"Go Dad Go!"
-Keaton St.Laurent, Jeffrey's eighteen-month-old son

"Jeffrey is a change agent. He is dynamic, motivating, and direct. This book is a must read for anyone wanting to create greater results in their life."

-Susan Sly, Author/success trainer
President and CEO of Step into Your Power Productions LLC

"Jeff is the epitome of Napoleon Hill fused with Arnold Schwarzenegger!"

-Scott Vautour, Student of Jeff's
and economics major at Harvard University

"Jeffrey cuts through all the noise going on in your head and compellingly delivers the bottom line of what is required from you to achieve fulfilling results in your life."

-Lois Tiedemann, Professional speaker/author,
www.TransformedTriathlete.com

"The unique perspective *Being Fulfilled* presents on what unlimited wealth is and how to attain it is spot on and ingenious. Jeff shares fresh ideas and original material that without a doubt will assist you with your results."

-Robert Cappuccio,
President and CEO of Legacy Performance Solutions

"Jeff St.Laurent leads a new generation of fantastic coaches that not only care about their clients, but avail themselves of all of the tools and technology available to retrain the mind and achieve maximum results. Being Fulfilled breaks down how to succeed and is chock-full of examples that inspire and motivate. I look forward to his next book!"

-Ridgely Goldsborough, Author of The Great Ones
www.AViewFromTheRidge.com

BEING
FULFILLED

Jeffrey St.Laurent

ISBN: 0-9740924-6-0

More Heart Than Talent Publishing, Inc.

6507 Pacific Ave #329
Stockton, CA 95207 USA
Toll Free: 800-208-2260
www.MHTPublishing.com

FAX: 209-467-3260

Cover art by FlowMotion Inc.

Printed in the United States of America

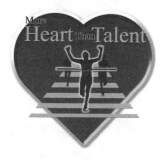

This book is dedicated to my wife, Jennifer, whom inspires me every day to grow and become better. Your honesty, integrity and love for us are what I cherish the most. Thank you for being my partner in so many ways.

TABLE OF CONTENTS

ACKNOWLEDGEMENTS   17

FOREWORD   25

A NOTE TO THE READER FROM THE AUTHOR   29

COACH'S CHALLENGE   33

SECTION I- A NEW MODEL FOR FULFILLMENT   35

What Is Unlimited Wealth?   35

A Model for Fulfillment   37

Never and Can't   42

A New Model for Fulfillment   44

Crème de la Business   48

Crème de la Relationships   49

Crème de la Health   50

I Wanna Be Like Mike   51

Focus Your Energy   53

The Why Behind How the Energy Points Are Allotted   58

"Most of Your Points" - Defined   61

"Most of Your Time" - Defined   62

How to Get Rid of Many Areas and Feel Okay   63

About Focus   65

The Big Picture   66

BEING FULFILLED

SECTION II– THE CORE STAGES AND PHILOSOPHIES   73

Seven Stages to Achieving Unlimited Wealth   73

Stage 1: Create a Vision   74

Stage 2: Simplify and Prioritize from that Vision   76

Stage 3: Structure and Organize Your Days around Your Priorities   78

Stage 4: Know Yourself and Establish Your New Rules   80

Stage 5: Find the Right People to Maintain the Focus
and Support the Vision   81

Stage 6: Maintain Focus *on that* Vision and *from that* Vision   82

Stage 7: Practice and Duplication   83

Ten Key Philosophies for Your Fulfillment   86

Philosophy #1: Embrace and Understand Change   86

Philosophy #2: Great Habits Produce Great Results   90

     How to Create a Habit   90

     The Sugar High   92

     Potential Barriers   95

     Four Steps to a New Habit   96

     Philosophy Summary   98

Coach's Challenge   **99**

Philosophy #3: Fulfillment Is Not a Matter of Circumstance;
It Is Largely a Matter of Conscious Choice   103

Philosophy #4: Results Are Energy   107

     How to Connect   108

     Energy Defined   111

     Trusting the Energy   112

     Becoming Attractive   113

     Attraction Is a Choice   117

     Coach's Challenge   **118**

Philosophy #5: When You Judge Yourself Less and Trust More
You Will Have Everything You Want   121

Philosophy #6: Perfection Does Not Exist   126

TABLE OF CONTENTS

Philosophy #7: Fear of Success Is Greater than Fear of Failure   129
    Let's Get Honest, Fear Is Not the Cause   131
    Why People Procrastinate and Sabotage their Progress   132
Philosophy #8: Balance as You Know It Does Not Exist
    and Is Not Necessary   136
Philosophy #9: Become Focused, Not Busy   139
Philosophy #10: Act Before You Think   140
What's Next?   146

SECTION III – THE SEVEN STAGES APPLIED TO BUSINESS   147

How to Achieve Unlimited Wealth via Business   147
The Seven Stages   150
Stage 1: Create a Business Vision   150
    How to Create a Clear and Certain Business Vision   152
Stage 2: Simplify and Prioritize from that Vision   155
    Seven Steps on How to Simplify and Prioritize from Your
    Business Vision   157
Stage 3: Structure and Organize Your Days around Your Priorities 162
    Six Steps to Structure and Organize Your Day   164
Stage 4: Know Yourself and Establish Your New Rules   173
    Three Steps to Understand Yourself, Your Rules
    … and Change!   177
Stage 5: Find the Right People to Maintain the Focus and
    Support the Vision   182
Stage 6: Maintain Focus *on that* Vision and *from that* Vision   191
Stage 7: Practice and Duplication   194
What's Next?   196

SECTION IV – THE SEVEN STAGES APPLIED TO RELATIONSHIPS   197

How to Achieve Unlimited Wealth via Relationships   197
Relationship Defined   197
Potential Barriers to Fulfillment   199

BEING FULFILLED

Are You Ready for a Fulfilling Relationship?   201

The Seven Stages   205

Stage 1: Create a Relationship Vision   205

     How to Create a Clear and Certain Relationship Vision   207

Stage 2: Simplify and Prioritize from that Vision   211

     Seven Steps on How to Simplify & Prioritize
from Your Relationship Vision   213

Stage 3: Structure and Organize Your Days around Your Priorities   217

     Six Steps to Structure and Organize Your Day   217

Stage 4: Know Yourself and Establish your New Rules   221

     Three Steps to Understand Yourself, Your Rules…
and Change!   221

Stage 5: Find the Right Person to Maintain the Focus
and Support the Vision   227

Stage 6: Maintain Focus *on that* Vision and *from that* Vision   234

Stage 7: Practice and Duplication   236

What's Next?   237

SECTION V – THE SEVEN STAGES APPLIED TO HEALTH   239

How to Achieve Unlimited Wealth via Health   239

The Fitness - Wealth Connection   239

True Health - The Backbone of Wealth   241

Jeff's Law of Wealth   242

Your Health Focus   244

The Seven Stages   247

Stage 1: Create a Health Vision   247

How to Create a Clear and Certain Health Vision   249

Stage 2: Simplify and Prioritize from that Vision   253

     Seven Steps on How to Simplify and Prioritize
from Your Health Vision   254

Stage 3: Structure and Organize Your Days around Your Priorities   259

     Six Steps to Structure and Organize Your Day   260

TABLE OF CONTENTS

Stage 4: Know Yourself and Establish Your New Rules   265
    Three Steps to Understand Yourself, Your Rules
    … and Change!   268
Stage 5: Find the Right People to Maintain the Focus and Support
    the Vision   274
Stage 6: Maintain Focus *on that* Vision and *from that* Vision   279
Stage 7: Practice and Duplication   282
What's Next?   285

SECTION VI – BETTER BODY, BIGGER BUCKS   287

Health Equity   290
Common Mindset   292
Your Money *IS* Where Your Mouth Is   294
What You Intuitively Know But Don't Want to Hear   298
Coach's Challenge   302
Your Path to a Better Body Bigger Bucks- "Jeff's Experiment"   306
Coach's Challenge   309
Beer-Gut Mentality   312
What's Next?   313

SECTION VII – MULTIPLE STREAMS OF FITNESS   315

Dive into the Lake of Fitness   317
Multiple Streams of Nutrition   319
The Energy of Nutrition   322
Multiple Streams of Exercise   323
Residual Muscle **Income**   326
If You are Easily Offended, Don't Read This   330

WHERE DO WE GROW FROM HERE?   333
THE BEGINNING   334
ABOUT THE AUTHOR   335
RESOURCES   337

BEING FULFILLED

ACKNOWLEDGEMENTS

Success is sweet. Success is even sweeter and far more extraordinary when you have a team of incredible people on your side. I am fortunate in my life to be surrounded with incredible people that inspire, encourage, and support my wild and crazy ideas and high energy visions. I am a person of trust, integrity, and honor, and I only surround myself with people that are the same. In my journey I have connected with many people that I learned from and trust explicitly. To the people below and everyone else not mentioned, I send my warmest thanks and gratitude. I look forward to the exciting future that we are creating together and look forward to basking in our glory high on the mountain of fulfillment!

To all my personal training clients and group fitness participants who have trusted me with their health and looked to me for support, motivation, and accountability, know how I appreciate all you have provided me with—most importantly, your dedication and commitment to yourself.

This book was partially written from my own experiences in life and business. However, what really made it possible were the thousands of hours I have invested with my personal coaching clients. You trusted me and yourself enough to share the deepest and most intimate experiences of your life, to place fear aside, and jump on the cold hard road of action.

Every session is as much a breakthrough for me as it is for you. My content and philosophies throughout this book were derived mainly from the notes I took from each and every session we shared. This book is yours; you wrote it, and you deserve the best life has to offer and all you are willing to create.

To Melanie Patterson, who of all my clients as of this writing has the award for fearlessness. You have inspired me to become a better coach and expect more from myself and other clients. Thanks for your bravery and for connecting me with some incredible people to endorse my book.

My passion for finding a way to empower people to create sustained results via their own strengths and values began when I attended The Institute for Professional Empowerment Coaching (iPEC). To all my teachers and classmates, you ignited a flame inside me for coaching that will never be extinguished. I want to especially thank Bruce D. Schneider, who was the catalyst in my coaching career. I respect all you have done and what you and your school represent to the world. The powers you possess have truly been a guiding force in my life and career.

To my mentor and coach, Jeffrey Combs, words cannot express what you have assisted me in creating. I respect you and what you do in more ways than can be expressed. You are responsible for allowing me to trust on a deeper level. I can honestly say that if I did not work with you, listen to, and more importantly, take action on everything you told me to, I would not be in the position I am today, and this book would not exist. Your information and workshop Breakthroughs to Success has allowed me a new level of success. Everyone deserves to experience all you and Erica have to offer. I also want to send the warmest thanks to Erica Combs, who has truly shown me what it is like to be in your power. I have seen you develop so much over the last few years, and you constantly impress me with your amazing insights. It has been a pleasure collaborating with you in the development of my first book and I look forward to more!

There is an amazing company out there called Body Training Systems that I have been involved with in many different capacities since 1998, when I first was trained as a group fitness instructor. Through my involvement with them I have had some of the greatest opportunities in the fitness industry that any fitness professional could aspire to dream of. There are so many fellow trainers and staff that I owe heaps of gratitude and thanks for shaping and molding me into the trainer and presenter I am today. There is one woman by the name of Cathy Spencer Browning who above all has influenced my life greatly… thank you for believing in a young, naïve, and passionate boy. You took me in and literally molded me into the strong, powerful, confident, and impactful man that I am today.

Many years ago when I graduated from college, I met John and Cathy Bonica who allowed me my first opportunities in the fitness industry. Since 1998 have I have witnessed firsthand what it truly takes to succeed in the health and fitness industry from behind the scenes. I thank you both most for believing in me as I began my wonderful journey in fitness and all your support along the way.

I have had a lot of role models in my life. One key role model for me was Peg Gorman, who I first met as one of her personal training clients. I was twenty-five and she was sixty-five. She became a friend of mine (though she will admit I was her "boy toy!"). At the time I was in a relationship but was not as fulfilled as I knew I could be. This is where Peg became my relationship role model. If there were a perfect

19

relationship, Peg had it. I admired her so much I included an interview with her on my audio course: Healthy Mind, Healthy Body, which has strengthened hundreds of relationships of listeners all around the world. Thanks for teaching me what true love is and showing me how to cherish every moment that I have.

When I became a dad I was so thrilled, and I had a fierce desire to be the best I could. My great friend Rex Repaire became my father role model. Ask anybody what Rex is great at… they will first and foremost say he is a great dad. Rex, thanks for not only inspiring me to become a better trainer and presenter, but more importantly, for showing me how to be a great dad.

I want to send my heartfelt thanks to my cousin, Michael Debitetto. You defined me as a teenager and truly taught me what it was like to be an entrepreneur. You gave me my eye for detail and quality. You showed me the discipline of hard work and consistency. You allowed me to feel what it was like to work hard and reap the financial rewards of being an entrepreneur. I would not be as successful as I am today or have the disciplines and habits necessary to succeed in business if it were not for your guidance, support, and unconditional love.

It is very rare in life that we are able to meet another person who shares so many of the same visions, passions, and values that you possess; a person who you instantly connect with and know from that moment on, you will collaborate with for a lifetime. That woman is Patty Abraham. Since we met, we have been kindred spirits and share an incredible vision of creating the life of our dreams, without compromise. Your business models, passion, and wisdom have allowed me to know even more certainly that I can and will create everything I have ever dreamed of. Thanks for the connections you have allowed me, the trust you have shown me, and the future you are assisting me in creating.

Special thanks go to Thomjon Borges, my marketing genius. The brand that we have created together will impact millions! Big thanks to Chris and Jamie Mattock of Flow Motion, Inc. who produced my audio course as well as the cover art and interior layout and design for this book. You are both the best at your craft, and I consider you my friends. To Claudia Volkman, my editor, who was able to take my thoughts and ideas and turn them into understandable sentences! While I was reading the first round of edits I was truly amazed at how you were able to make my own words make even more sense to me! Thank you for your skills and wisdom.

I cannot forget my boys… my strong friends that will be there forever. Mark Boldeia, you have known me the longest and no matter where life takes us, the memories we have created will stay with us forever. You are the person I can talk to about anything, and I cherish that. Gregg Rivinius, you and I have seen and shared so much together as college roommates. The college days and memories will keep us connected forever. Thanks for the great times and more to come. Jeffrey Mielke, from college to the present, you are a sounding board, a prankster, my eternal rival in billiards, my web designer, my tech guy, future movie producer, and best of all… an incredible friend. I look forward to fifty years down the road shooting billiards and sharing great stories. Patrick Lyden, you are someone who came into my life when I was not taking any more applications for friends. We have shared many common interests and passions since and have a great connection. You inspire me to compete at a higher level on and off the bike. I cannot wait to be a dad together, hike again, talk business, and drop your ass when we ride! Of course, I cannot leave out Angela Lyden who not only makes a great "rabbit" when we ride, but is my junk food eating buddy!

I am not sure if any one has ever included their dog in the acknowledgements, but I am more than happy to be the first. Cosmo, even though you will never read this, you know every day how much I love your unending support. You sat at my feet and licked my feet as I wrote this book into the wee hours of the night. You have shown me what unconditional love is and how to not let other people's bad moods impact your day. You have shown me how always wanting to play and run is okay and the more you do it the better you feel. You have taught me how to laugh even more and have provided much stress relief when you lick my face or jump up and tackle me.

To Keaton, my incredibly adorable son... oh, how you have taught me how to love on a deeper level than I ever dreamed possible. When you are old enough to read this, let's spend a weekend alone together so I can share how you have empowered me to live, love, and laugh on a higher plane.

Thanks to my mother-in-law, Diana Cleland Boyle, who has been one of my biggest fans. I must thank you for raising an incredible daughter whom I adore more than life itself. You have shown me love in so many ways, but most of all by showing genuine interest in all my passions by listening to me and sharing amazing insights to life and business that I value greatly. You ground me when necessary and have assisted me in more ways than I can express.

ACKNOWLEDGEMENTS

To Steven, my "little" brother who still thinks he is taller than me. Even though you are, in fact, taller, I am still most proud to be your "big" brother. The memories we have shared could fill a whole book, and I look forward to filling many more together. If there is someone that I can count on and trust with my life, you are the one. Of all the things you have taught me, having 100% faith is the biggest. Your faith has brought you so much reward in life, and you have allowed me to leap off bigger mountains fearless and faithful.

To my sister-in-law, Cathy, thank you for being my "sister." I have always wanted a sister, and you are the one and only. Thanks for making my brother so happy and being the one and only perfect person for him. I am so thrilled you found each other. I especially want to thank you for the great drawings and figures you drew for my first book. I love that you have contributed to this passion of mine.

Dad, what more can I say than thanks for being the world's greatest dad in my book! You have instilled in me more than you can ever know. I hope you take great pride in knowing that my success is a direct reflection of your discipline, love, hard work, sacrifice, and guidance you have instilled in me over my lifetime. I am so proud of what you have accomplished in your life and am excited to see you enjoy the next phase of your life. There is not a day that passes that I am not thinking about you or striving to be as solid, consistent, and successful as you are. Continue to take great care of yourself so we can share many more years of love together.

Okay, Mom, if my eyes are watering while I am writing this, you better get some tissues out. I dedicate my success in life to my #1 teacher: MOM. From changing diapers to staying up all night helping with my fourth grade "Florida" project that I forgot about, to going out of your way to help me with anything I ask of you... thank you for your unconditional love. You have raised me to be smart, successful, caring, and filled with love for life. You have shown me what it is to be a survivor against the worst odds. You are the strongest person I know, and every day for the rest of my life I will aspire to possess that quality. Seeing the way you adore my son as a grandmother, has brought a newfound, deeper love and appreciation for what you have done for me and the caring you gave me and still do today. Take care of yourself, because I have big plans for us!

To Jennifer... my soul mate, lover, best friend, training partner, teammate, wife, and mother of my son... I will always adore you. Alone, I am great... with you, I am world class and beyond. Any words I write are minuscule compared to the genuine passion I possess deep in my soul for our love. There is only one person for each of us, and you are the one for me. There is only one thing that I love more than you... US, I love us. Cheers to JJ Forever.

FOREWORD

In our world, some things occur as natural laws of the universe: gravity works no matter where you live; humans need oxygen in order to survive; and no matter how many things you place on your to-do list, there are only twenty-four hours in each day.

Although it's not a natural law, another universal idea is that most of us live our lives wanting to feel "more fulfilled." We know what that means and how that might feel, but the method of how we achieve that sense is absent. In *Being Fulfilled,* Jeffrey St. Laurent presents a model which challenges the conventional way of thinking and helps us fill in the gap between wanting more and actually enjoying more.

Most readers start this book *thinking* about how their lives would look if they were fulfilled. But therein lies a problem: In life, we achieve the feeling of being fulfilled by *feeling*, not thinking. Thinking is a logical step in the process of becoming more fulfilled. The act of being fulfilled, however, is a feeling of inspiration, joy, peace, and satisfaction. These feelings come from our heart, not our head. The insights and examples in *Being Fulfilled* will escort readers from thinking about being fulfilled to ultimately *feeling* more fulfilled.

BEING FULFILLED

Chances are, if you were somewhat drawn to the title and actually picked up this book, you are someone who lives with big dreams and visions. Though dreams and visions are admirable, some visions are so broad that they are unattainable.

Being Fulfilled teaches you how to change your patterns of thought and actually live the life you dream about. Jeffrey helps us narrow our vision and then focus, nurture, and train in ONE area. Once we learn these techniques for one area, we can dramatically enrich the three most significant areas of life: business, relationships, and health.

Imagine that you are a champion thoroughbred horse preparing for a race. The important components of your success lie in your talent, training, passion, and ability to focus. To improve your chances for victory, you even wear blinders to help restrict the vision of everything going on around you. With this narrowed vision, you are purely focused on your goal. When it comes to leading a more fulfilled life, Jeffrey suggests that you "put the blinders on" and offers a step-by-step guide to assist you in achieving your vision.

As a motivational speaker, life coach, and author, Jeffrey is talented, curious, and questions the ordinary. For example, in *Being Fulfilled*, Jeffrey questions the idea that there IS a magical point on which to stand where business, relationships, and health are in perfect harmony. With millions of people searching for this magnificent, yet somewhat fabricated place, wouldn't it be helpful if we directed our efforts to an authentic destination?

When people meet Jeffrey St. Laurent, they struggle to fully describe his uniqueness, professionalism, sensitivity, personal power, integrity, brilliance, and puppy-like playfulness. What is now a human magnet to greatness was once a person unaware of his power and potential. To see Jeffrey speak at a workshop or in front of a group fitness class, it's hard to believe that he spent many years of his life being quiet, insecure, overweight, sensitive, and naïve. Though some of those qualities are still part of him, he's learned to use them to benefit his life and the lives of those around him.

Most authors have great ideas. In order for their ideas transform someone's life, however, an author has to tickle our imagination in a way that makes the ideas go from something we think about to something we believe in. In *Being Fulfilled*, Jeffrey is lively and straight to the point as he reveals his secrets of how to live your life with more joy and satisfaction.

From the moment I met Jeffrey St. Laurent, I was "wowed" by his uniqueness, insights, and understanding. After reading *Being Fulfilled*, my guess is you will nod your head in agreement with my opinion that he is truly exceptional, extremely talented, and a person who has the ability to improve your life in many ways. I am proud to say he is a great influence in my life and has helped make many of my dreams come true. I wish you the best in your journey of *Being Fulfilled*.

Jennifer Hoy St. Laurent
Certified life coach, motivational speaker,
& proud wife of Jeffrey St. Laurent

www.SweetSpotCoach.com

BEING FULFILLED

A NOTE
TO THE READER
FROM THE AUTHOR

I am sitting in the middle of the woods on a big cold rock. My lips are chapped from the cold November air as I type these words onto my lap top. My dog, Cosmo, is running circles around me grabbing sticks, jumping in and out of the mud and swimming in the lake that is just off to my left. He runs by me and sprays mud all over me and my lap top. I try and wipe the mud and water off the screen with my glove but it smears the mud more.

I walked through the woods to get to this place. This is a beautiful place just behind my house up over the hill. It is a calm place at the entrance to a forest where there is a running stream that flows into a lake with beautiful scenery which sooths and calls me to an inner peace.

I consider this to be more than just a physical place; it is a state of being. This is a place inside my heart I call fulfillment.

As I type these words, the book you are about to read has been written, edited and ready to print. It is a book about *being fulfilled* and how you can arrive at that wonderful place… a feeling of completeness, peace and serenity. Fulfillment is a place where I have been before and constantly strive to be. The ironic part of this whole situation and the very nature of my writing this to you is that currently I am not as fulfilled as I would like to be.

I write this only to be honest and open. You deserve that. I have had many challenges in life, have grown tremendously from them and continue to do so. This book is another step in that journey. My intent with this book and what I just shared is to paint a realistic picture of what fulfillment possibly is and a promising method of achieving it. I would be lying if I said everything was perfect. I would be fooling you if I painted a picture of this magical place like in the forest and said it was easy to get there.

So what is fulfillment? That is something that you will have to define for yourself and this book will assist you with doing so. What I want to express here is that from what I understand, fulfillment is a moving target. You can feel fulfilled one moment and realize it's gone in the next. Fulfillment is something we are and will be constantly striving for. Your efforts in *being fulfilled* will never end.

I don't write this book because I am the fulfillment expert or I am supposed to tell you what to do. I don't write this because I am completely fulfilled and always will be. I write this rather to show you that there is hope and possibility. I write this to be candid and real so that you can release the pressures you and society have placed upon yourself. The philosophies and stages in this book are real and tested. They have delivered much fulfillment in my life in many areas at different times. That being said, the reality is, in a moment, in a choice or with a single thought... all of that can go away.

When fulfillment goes away, it can feel like there is no hope or worth left in my world.

But the book calls me to stand up and get real. I am getting real with you and sharing this because I know that it is the most difficult thing for me to do. I also know that speaking my deep truth is where fulfillment lies... on the other side of the most difficult choices. The challenge is to acknowledge that in my moments of decision, when deep down inside I know what is right and moral, I am sometimes scared to take the high road. Unlimited fulfillment demands my honesty, trust and courage.

I have taken the high road many times and know the low road quite well. Even with all my expertise and experience... to this day I still have trouble choosing the high road. When fear knocks on my door, I am no different than anyone else. Some days I will have the courage and choose the high road and other days... I will falter to my addictions and poor habits and be far less than I ever wanted to be. This is real; this is where releasing the true truth will set you on the road to fulfillment.

I have learned that there is the truth and then the true truth. The truth is what you know to be true through *your* reality. I have seen that my reality...in reality...can sometimes be a lie. The true truth is a place where you can put aside (usually with the assistance of others) all the excuses and stop rationalizing (rational lies). This will then expose a situation or reality that will present you with two choices... the high or low road. The high road WILL be the most difficult to choose and WILL ultimately lead you to fulfillment. The major question is... which will you choose?

I look forward to seeing you on the road to *being fulfilled.*

Jeffrey St.Laurent

BEING FULFILLED

COACH'S CHALLENGE

Throughout this book, you will see several sections with a Coach's Challenge. Each challenge is purposefully designed to utilize the information delivered in that section and assist you with facilitating action. Understand each challenge will allow your results to be greater. These are specifically designed to stimulate the mind-body connection and reprogram your old patterns that keep you doing the same thing over and over.

The further objective of these tested challenges is to develop new behaviors conducive to bigger results. They are very ritualistic in nature and may have you doing things out of the ordinary. In order to develop new behavior patterns and habits, you must be stimulated, using all of your senses. Some examples are seeing something different in your environment, speaking different words out loud, hearing different messages from yourself and your environment, smelling unique scents that remind you of something new and exciting, or feeling new sensations that stimulate empowering emotions

I purposely included different challenges for different types of people. We all learn, process, and digest information differently. These challenges have had great success when used on myself and my clients. I include them, because they are tested and *will work* when you invest the time. If you are having trouble working through some of the challenges or want to really maximize them, see the back of the book for information on our phenomenal *Being Fulfilled* nine-week coaching experience.

SECTION I

A NEW MODEL
FOR FULFILLMENT

What Is Unlimited Wealth?

When you think of "wealth," what ideas, thoughts, and feelings come to mind? Do you think of money, traveling, time off, and the ability to buy more expensive goods and services? The objective of this book is to broaden your perspective on wealth. When you expand your perspective on wealth, your whole life can change.

Before we go any further, we must first define the term wealth. As a life coach, I often hear my clients say that they want to be more successful, wealthier, happier, more fulfilled, more physically fit, etc. Before achieving excellence in any area of life, the end result must be clear and well-defined. Though many people seek to "be wealthy," many have not taken the time to express what "being wealthy" means in words. That being said, what is your definition of wealth? Write your definition below.

My definition of wealth is:_____

_____

_____

BEING FULFILLED

If we compared your definition to one hundred other readers, you would see one hundred different answers. There might be a common theme, such as having a lot of money, taking a break, spending more time with friends, and something to do with owning luxurious personal possessions. In *Being Fulfilled,* we will propose a new look at the term wealth and how feeling wealthy, in this sense, can change your life

Recently I did a survey and asked fifty clients to define wealth. Ninety-five percent of them included money as the main component of wealth. Money is definitely an element of wealth. But when you appreciate "unlimited wealth," money is no longer the only ingredient. When you look at getting rich financially, money is what you need to fulfill your goal. But if your goal is to achieve unlimited wealth, I challenge you to look beyond the money. I was brought up hearing that money is not everything. Agreed. Money is *not everything;* however, it is *a part* of everything. So, what is wealth? One client answered: "Wealth is having *it* all!" It... It... What is "It"?

I am going to propose that wealth is something not tangible at all. It's not something you can buy or hold, but rather a feeling. Wealth is a feeling where you have an inner sense of fulfillment. Even though we have all felt a sense of fulfillment, the majority of us don't hold that feeling permanently. Most people live on an emotional wave that goes in and out of fulfillment like they are doing the Hokey Pokey.

The reason for this is that people do not know how to duplicate their fulfillment from one area to the next. The average person can achieve something great and still not know exactly how they got there. They quickly celebrate and then move on to their next "to do." What would happen if you reached a new level of fulfillment, and then took the time to examine how you got there? What if you discovered a way to duplicate the way you became fulfilled? In other words, *what if you could create an actual process with steps and guidelines that not only would allow you to feel more fulfilled, but would teach you how to get there again should you lose the feeling?*

That is **exactly** what this book will teach you to do! By the time you finish this book, you will have learned a results tested and proven process that you can run yourself through anytime to not only feel fulfilled, but sustain that feeling long-term in *all* areas of your life! This is what we call unlimited wealth. **Unlimited wealth is a complete, duplicatable, sustained feeling of fulfillment in all areas of your life.**

A Model for Fulfillment

When I think of all the areas of my life and what it would take to attain complete fulfillment in these areas, I get overwhelmed. How *do* you attain complete fulfillment in *all* areas? Is it possible to grow and maintain a business, be part of a family, raise children, be in love, socialize with friends, maintain a household, pay bills, save for retirement, create wise investments, exercise, eat well, improve your fitness, travel, live life to its fullest, have fun with your hobbies, have down time, have time to reflect on the spiritual side of living, shop, balance your checkbook, balance your life, and make your bed every morning? Is it possible to maintain balance and attain unlimited wealth without being neurotic?

The following is a model for fulfillment called the Wheel of Life. As you can see in Figure A, it is essentially a circle divided into eight pieces.

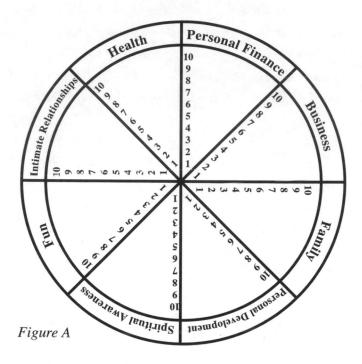

Figure A

You divide your life into eight different categories and write each category on the wheel. The wheel's eight categories are:

1) Family

2) Personal Development

3) Spiritual Awareness

4) Fun

5) Intimate Relationships

6) Health

7) Personal Finance

8) Business

For each section of the wheel, circle your *current* level of fulfillment in that area using the number scale. The higher the number (ten being the highest), the more fulfilled you are in that area. The lower the number (one being the lowest), the less fulfilled you are. After circling a number in each category, connect the adjacent numbers. In other words, take your pen and put it on the number you circled in Personal Development and draw a line straight across to the number you circled in the Spiritual Awareness. Do this with all eight categories. When you connect all your circles, what shape is your wheel? For example, notice on Figure B, this person circled a perfect ten in all eight categories. This shape makes a nice, round wheel, doesn't it? If this wheel represented how you live your life, you would be rolling along smoothly, right?

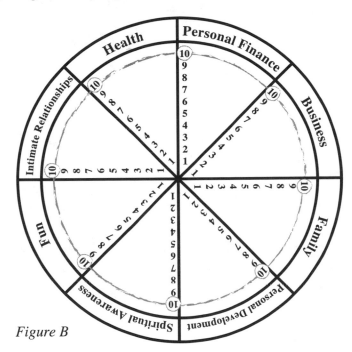

Figure B

Notice on Figure C this person circled a more realistic snapshot of their life. If this shapely wheel represented your life, how would it roll? Would it be a bumpy journey? Exactly!

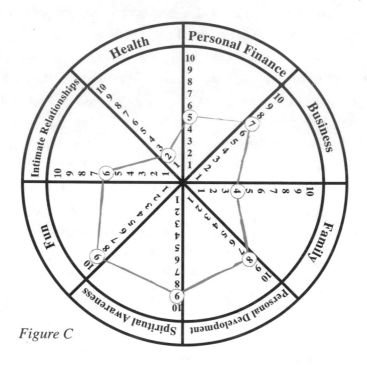

Figure C

The Wheel of Life is a great tool to quickly identify an area of your life that might require your attention so things "roll" smoother. For example, let's say I rate myself an eight (or above) in all categories except business (which is a three). Based on my low rating in business, it's obvious I need to focus on improving my business. So, I commit and decide to focus on my company. After three months of working hard on my business, I revisit my wheel and re-rate myself in all eight categories. On my new rating, the business category improved significantly, but two of my other category ratings have dropped. This was not by choice. I didn't deliberately choose to let things go; it just happened. When I focused my attention on one area, that area improved. Regrettably, the others areas fell. This is not only a trend I experienced, it is one many others have encountered as well.

No matter how hard I work, it seems I cannot balance *every* category in my life and get them to a level nine or ten, which is where I want them to be. If I really focused and took bold action, I could get *one* category there, but not *all* of them at the same time. Complete fulfillment seems unrealistic. The idea of work-life balance is becoming an impossible dream. I am beginning to accept that my "wheel" will never be properly balanced or roll smoothly. I'm beginning to think my wheel would always resemble the shape of a starfish. The worst part is, those eight categories are not enough to describe my ideal life. By the time I was done with the wheel of life I wanted to create, I had about ten sub categories in each of the main categories. My wheel looked something like Figure D

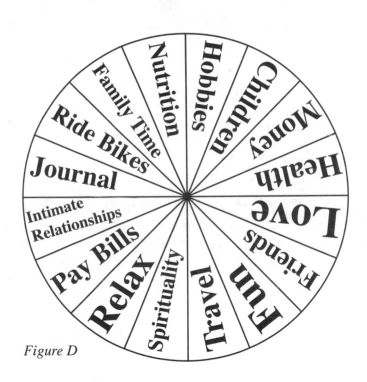

Figure D

Never and Can't

As a certified empowerment coach and motivational speaker, I encourage people to release the words *never* and *can't* from their vocabulary because they can be very limiting. The problem is, while we're striving for complete fulfillment, the words *never* and *can't* seem to ring loud and true. In my case, even though I worked through so much and achieved much success, I still felt I'd never achieve that feeling of unlimited wealth.

Throughout most of our lives, we've heard that we can be, do, and have everything we want. We're led to believe that we can *be* everything and be great *at* everything. We've heard philosophies like "it just takes time and patience" to reach our goals. We've heard that we can have everything if we just apply focus and passion.

As I explored my desire to be a successful entrepreneur, inspiring author, a loving husband and father, a competitive athlete, a friend and son who spent time with important people, I had a grand insight. What if the people who taught us those "rules" are wrong? What if I challenged everything I knew and tried a different way? What if it was impossible to be a ten in all areas of our life *at the same time?* If it were impossible, what would that mean? If it were impossible to get everything I wanted, how would I feel? What if the words "can't" and "never" *were* applicable here?

My conclusion and how I answered those questions was that, in my wheel of life I **CAN'T** be a ten in all areas **at once.** (Don't even think about trying to be an eight or nine either). I **never** will be 100% at the same time! No matter how hard I focus, no matter how much passion I apply, it's simply not going to happen. You can challenge it, rationalize it, disagree with it, or feel slightly discouraged at the idea. I'm not writing this to discourage you, but to give you a new perspective and help you face the reality of what one can be and do in a twenty-four-hour day.

Though reality is sometimes scary, when you embrace it, you are able to move forward into a place where you can produce better results. I have heard many stories of people who live in a state of dissatisfaction because of their "go, go, go" way of life. When one's way of thinking and their expectations are improbable, they finish their day feeling like there is still so much they want or have to do. Embracing those philosophies lead us to a constant state of disappointment. However, when we embrace the idea that it's impossible to be a ten in all areas of our life at the same time, we allow room for personal satisfaction and joy.

When I accepted the reality that being a perfect ten in all areas was impossible, I felt a big pressure being lifted from me. It was like an eight-ton elephant just stepped off my chest. When I admitted it was impossible, I felt like it was not my fault anymore and there was nothing wrong with me for not being able to achieve it. What a relief!

I consider myself to have great habits, unparalleled discipline, great health, an unshakable mindset, and a laser sharp focus. Even with all those qualities on my side, I still could not achieve this alluring balance that everyone talks about. What I realized is that I was not the only one feeling this way. In fact, everyone I coached, talked to, heard of, met, or read about was the same. Even the best success coaches, authors, and speakers had something missing at one point in their lives. No matter who we are, there was, or will be, some area less fulfilled than the others.

Even though I felt a little relief, I was still faced with the reality that I was unfulfilled in some areas of my life. I was still sick of having phases of my life where I felt great followed by times where I could barely breathe. Then I asked myself a question: What if complete fulfillment *was* possible but I was following the wrong rules and using the wrong model? Just because I could not be fulfilled in all areas *at once*, **what if I could be really fulfilled in one area without neglecting the others?**

In other words, what if I could be a ten in business and be a five in other areas, and actually feel fulfilled? Why do I have to be a ten in all areas to be fulfilled? What if there were too many areas that I was trying to be great at? What if my odds for success would be greater if I created a new model for fulfillment?

A New Model for Fulfillment

All these questions began to unlock a new vision. My vision was to create a new model for myself and my seminar participants and coaching clients that would allow a realistic avenue to achieve unlimited wealth.

This new model really took shape one day after I challenged a coaching client. She was talking about her life and her overwhelming responsibilities. She said, "It is tough to fit it all in." I said, "Why do you have to fit it all in?" She did not have a really good answer to that, and neither did I. This challenge opened a new shift in thinking: Why is it that we feel we have to fit it all in? What are all the things you're trying to fit in? More importantly, *why* are you trying to fit more in?

What would happen if you dropped the mindset of thinking that you needed to be great at everything today? What would happen if you gave yourself permission to be great in certain areas at certain times, but not in *all* areas at *all* times? When I gave myself permission to not fit everything in, I asked myself, what did I *want* to fit in? My immediate answer was everything! After laughing at my "wanting it all" rituals and habits of the past, I began to focus on the areas I really wanted to make an impact on.

I took an honest look at how I achieved fulfillment in the past. The process for achieving fulfillment in each area boiled down to the same formula: consistent laser focus with repetitive, productive action over a long period of time (years). The real key is consistent laser focus with repetitive, productive action over a long period of time… **in ONE AREA.** The only way you might be able to focus on *two* areas is if you are single and have no intimate relationship to speak of. If you are like most people in a serious, intimate relationship, married, with children and other big responsibilities, **one area of focus is the limit in any one time frame.**

As I began to look at my wheel of life with my eight categories and my other eighty sub-categories, I began to feel a bit lost. I understood the value of focusing on one area, but what about the others? If I focused on my business, did that mean my relationships, health, and all the other areas had to suffer and go downhill? Didn't that defeat the purpose? How would focusing on only one area really allow me to attain unlimited wealth? How could I only focus on one area when I had so many that I wanted and needed to focus on?

This is when I challenged the wheel of life with all its categories, tore it up, and decided it needed to be simplified. I came up with a new model seen in Figure E. As seen in this figure, for simplicity's sake unlimited wealth breaks down into three main categories: Business, Relationships, and Health. Unlimited wealth is the overall fulfillment from a combination of these three categories. Let's toss out all the other categories we can think of. I recognize there is religion, spirituality, social and personal growth, and a whole lot more. But for the sake of those businessmen and women, entrepreneurs and career-driven readers, I am using these three areas that are the most profitable and attainable ways of fulfillment in your life.

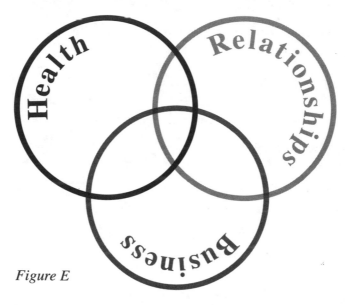

Figure E

While the three categories *can* stand on their own, it is important to recognize how they are very connected and dependent on each other when it comes to attaining unlimited wealth. In addition, how you attain complete fulfillment in each area, as you will soon see, is strikingly the same.

Let's look at three people in different situations to better see how each category depends on each of the others to attain the unlimited wealth I speak of.

Person One: *If you asked a millionaire woman who has a profitable business but just lost the love of her life if she feels wealthy, what would she say?*

Person Two: *If you asked a man who is super fit, in great health, but flat out broke if he feels wealthy, what would he say?*

Person Three: *If you asked anyone who has all the money in the world but is laid up in a hospital bed if they feel wealthy, what would they say?*

The first person has a great business but no relationship. The second person has great health but no business. The last person has a great business but no health. It is clear to see that each category, in some capacity, depends on the other to create unlimited wealth.

Let me state some facts to see what we have established so far with this new model for fulfillment in business, relationships, and health.

- *Each category depends on the other.*
- *In order to be truly great in any category, you must have consistent laser focus with   repetitive,   productive action over a long period of time… in ONE AREA.*
- *While focusing on that one area, you must not feel like you are neglecting the other two.*
- *Remind yourself, "I can only be great in one area at any one time."*

Before we go any further, I want to explain clearly why someone can only be great in one area at a time. I'll explain the difference between someone who has unlimited wealth and someone who does not. I believe that we are all fundamentally the same; nobody is better than anyone else.

While we may have been cut from different cloths, at the end of the day we are all still cloth. If we are all fundamentally the same, what is the difference between someone who has unlimited wealth and someone who does not? Let's break down each category to see statistically who is in the top percentage, and what makes them different.

Crème de la Business

When it comes to defining success and fulfillment in business, the definitions can be widely varied, to say the least. I am going to define success and fulfillment here as the amount of income you earn from your business. Let's not even talk about profit, but simply income. At the end of the day, you can have all the fun in the world with what you do, but if you are not bringing home the bacon, how fulfilled can you really be? When you live paycheck to paycheck, unable to buy something you really want *or* need, constantly worrying about money and depriving yourself of experiences that require money, that is not fulfillment.

In business, ninety-seven percent of the population works for three percent of the population. About five percent of the population earns a six-figure income or more. One twentieth of one percent—yes, that's 1/20th of 1%—earns a seven-figure income or more. For some reason, entrepreneurs and business people have a sense of success and accomplishment that goes along with earning a six-figure income. According to the statistics, they should! Statistically, that would put them in the top five percent of the population.

What does it take to be in the top five percent of income-earners? People in the top five percent have different habits, motives, principles, and mindsets. So what is the common thread among them all? From my research of studying, being mentored, coaching, and learning from successful entrepreneurs, the one thread that is common among the top income earners is their ability to FOCUS ON ONE AREA, their business, for a long period of time. They eliminate other components of their life, either completely or partially, in order to focus on their business.

Crème de la Relationships

When it comes to defining success in relationships, the definitions, once again, are widely varied. I define success here as the constant feeling of being significant and adored by another person... hence the term "significant other." I believe that great relationships are in our lives to magnify our experiences and create a greater sense of fulfillment and worth. Great relationships magnify life's experiences much more than if we were alone.

With the percentage of couples getting divorced and breaking up these days, I began to wonder how fulfilled people really are with their current relationships. If you asked one hundred couples how fulfilled and completely satisfied they were in their relationships, what would they say? In an environment that is safe, open, and nonjudgmental, about five percent would answer that they are completely fulfilled. What about the other ninety-five percent? Just because they are not completely fulfilled does not mean they are in a bad relationship. Not rating their relationship at one hundred percent complete fulfillment just means they are not where they would like to be, and they must do something about it or nothing will change.

What does it take to be in the top five percent of the population in a relationship? We all know that people in the top five percent have similar morals, values, and dreams, but what is the common thread among them all? With every completely fulfilled couple I have coached or spoken to, the one thread common among them all is their ability to FOCUS ON ONE AREA, their relationship, for a long period of time. They too, eliminated other components of their life, either completely or partially, in order to focus on their relationship.

Crème de la Health

When it comes to fitness, sadly, eighty-five percent of the population does not meet the minimum standard for a healthy heart reported by the surgeon general. Years ago, the surgeon general report stated that for a healthy heart, one must exercise a minimum of thirty minutes, three times a week. Since then, the typical person's lifestyle has become more sedentary. With all the drive-up conveniences, elevators, escalators, computers, faxes, and phones, we can easily get through our entire day simply sitting.

Although our current lifestyle is easier than it was back in farming days, it's not necessarily better for our health. For example, look at diabetes: Type II diabetes was formerly labeled *adult onset diabetes*; now it is only called Type II diabetes because inactive and obese children are getting it. The modern mindset and convenient lifestyle have definitely changed our nation into a more sedentary population. Due to this devastating situation, the surgeon general has increased the exercise recommendation to a minimum of sixty minutes, seven days a week! And remember, that's the *minimum* standard to promote a healthy heart.

Let's take a closer look at the eighty-five percent that does not meet the minimum standard for a healthy heart. Sixty percent of that group does not achieve the recommended amount of regular physical activity required to stay healthy. The remaining twenty-five percent is completely inactive. That leaves fifteen percent of the population that exercises regularly. Of that fifteen percent, what percent would consider themselves, by their own definition, fulfilled with their current level of fitness? After being in the fitness industry since 1996, it is no shock to me that roughly five percent of regular exercisers are actually happy with their results.

What does it take to be in the top five percent of the healthy population? It is obvious that people in the top five percent have great discipline, great habits, and a high self-esteem. But what is the common thread among them all? You might have guessed that it is their ability to FOCUS ON ONE AREA, their health, for a long period of time. They too eliminated other components of their life, either completely or partially, to focus on their health.

I Wanna Be Like Mike

Based on what you just read in the three areas of business, relationships, and health, it seems that five percent of our population has trained themselves to focus on one area for a long period of time. **Your ability to focus in one area for a long period of time is the number one ingredient to achieving unlimited wealth**. You don't need skills or require talent. What you absolutely must possess is long-term focus in one area.

For example, take my twenty-five year old friend, Mike. Last year was his first year ever riding a road bike. Last year, he showed up at our Tuesday night club ride with his new bike and a big smile. These Tuesday night rides are very competitive and grueling, to say the least. The group is comprised of great athletes with years of cycling miles in their legs. Additionally, most of these cyclists are very competitive racers. When Mike showed up, we all introduced ourselves and learned that this was his first ride ever! We welcomed him to the group, but expressed the thought that he might want to ride with the beginner group, as our group rides fast. He shrugged his shoulders and said that he would be fine. About five miles into that fifty-mile ride, Mike was no where to be seen. He was, in cycling terms, "dropped!"

That did not stop Mike. Week after week, he showed up to the Tuesday night rides. Moreover, he rode several miles each week, in hopes of one day being strong enough to hang with this "A" group of riders. Each week Mike would hang with the group a little longer before being dropped.

The end of the cycling season in New England is defined by twenty degrees and three feet of snow covering the ground. With these conditions, cycling outdoors is not an option, even for the sickest of athletes. You have the option to wait until springtime to ride, or to put your bike on an indoor trainer, and spend the next five months pedaling indoors. Cycling on the indoor trainer can be incredibly boring, no matter what is in front of you. For that reason, most cyclists take those five months off from riding.

While all the other cyclists were gaining weight and taking a winter break, Mike kept up with his weekly training on his indoor trainer. At the first sign of spring, Mike was outside putting in some serious training time. By the first Tuesday night ride of next season, Mike came to the ride looking completely different. This season, he looked like a professional cyclist... arms like sticks and thighs like a V-12 engine. Five miles into the first ride, Mike was once again nowhere to be seen. This time, however, he did not get dropped—we did. Mike dropped the entire group! Mike made the entire group look like we had training wheels on our bikes.

In his second season, "rookie" Mike raced competitively and was finishing in the top ten. On several occasions, he placed in the top three with a podium finish. And that's not even the incredible part. Cycling races rate athletes in five categories: Category one, or pro, is the best; category five is where you begin. Mike began racing in category five. Within a few months, he was upgraded all the way up to category three! This is where he was putting in podium finishes! Everyone was asking Mike what his secret was. At the end of the day all of his success boiled down to the fact that he FOCUSED ON ONE AREA, cycling, for a long period of time (one year).

He maintained his relationship and kept his job, but his main focus for the majority of every day was to get faster on the bike. What was his result? He got faster on the bike. Mike did not have incredible skills, background, talent, or luck... all he did was focus on being great at one thing. You know the saying, "What you focus on grows?" The more focus you put on something, the more it grows. Okay, so now that it is clear that we must focus on one thing, the big question is not what do we focus *on*, but rather *what* do we focus?

Focus Your Energy

You deserve to find an easy way to focus your energy. In addition, you deserve to discover how to focus that energy in one area. We must be able to focus our energy because in any given day we only have so much emotional and physical energy to give. If you continually use more energy than you have, you'll burn out. When you try to do too much at one time, you end up "at the end of your rope" or "burning both ends of the candle." When you expend more energy than you have, exhaustion is bound to occur. Exhaustion also occurs when you have no focus at all. Both situations lend to individual burnout, frustration, and overwhelm.

Think of your daily energy as a debit card. The objective of a debit card is to use money you have—versus a credit card, which uses money you don't have. Each day, imagine you have ten dollars to put into this debit account. Let's refer to your ten dollars as ten energy points. Each day you must decide where you wish to invest these ten points of energy.

If you use more than ten points each day, you overdraw your account and begin to accrue debt. Think of this as a negative energy balance. If you have only ten points each day that you will definitely use, how can you ever get rid of the negative balance? This is how you accumulate energy debt. If you have an energy debt for too long, it *will* catch up with you, no matter how young and strong you think you are. The end result will leave you stressed and burnt-out.

Here is the reality of it: Each day, you need to expend all ten energy points somewhere. The scary part is, when you don't have a clear plan on how you'll invest these points, you'll end up accomplishing nothing and wasting them. This is typically when you *think* you need more resources and say things

> like "There is not enough time in the day," or "I need
> more money," or "I can never get anything done."
> The reality is that you do not require more resources,
> but rather the ability to focus the resources you do
> have.

Because we have a limited amount of energy to give, this new model for fulfillment states that, in any given day, we only possess ten points of energy. This energy can be wisely focused or carelessly spent. The following will teach you how to wisely and easily focus your precious energy to maximize your results. Look again at Figure D. Knowing you only have ten energy points to use each day, where do you put them?

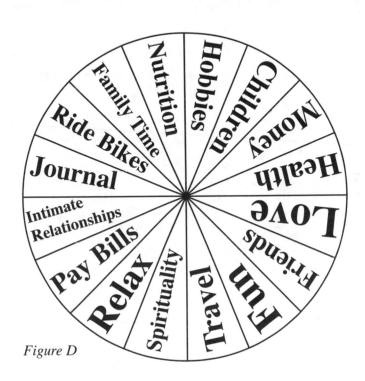

Figure D

When I tried to place my ten energy points on this wheel, I constantly wished for more points to distribute. As much as I yearned for more energy to work with each day, the bottom line is, those points were unobtainable. I don't have them and neither do you. I couldn't focus on being good at everything I wanted to be, do, and have. I couldn't start each day with the intent of being a good son, instructor, businessman, friend, athlete, spiritual leader, grow my career, make sure my house and car were perfectly clean, and eat good foods throughout the day. No matter how hard I tried, I could not be good in each of those areas every single day. Moreover, I did not want to be "good"... I wanted to be great! As I said earlier, the only way one can be great is by focusing on one area for a long period of time.

So I scratched the thirty categories in the old wheel of life and brought in the new unlimited wealth model for fulfillment. This new model defines unlimited wealth as an overall fulfillment from a combination of three categories: business, relationships, and health. Knowing that the only way I can be great is by focusing most of my energy in one of these three areas for a long period of time, I needed to determine how much of my ten energy points each day I could allot in one area that would actually produce a great result. Let's say I wanted to focus on growing a profitable business. I tried distributing my energy points like this:

Business	Relationship	Health
4	3	3

When I divided my points "equally," it kept me feeling
- *Average in all three areas and, ironically, never balanced*
- *Like I couldn't gain much progress in any one area*
- *Frustrated and spread out*
- *Like I was never focused on any one specific area*
- *Unfulfilled*

So then I tried a different way to grow a profitable business.

Business	Relationship	Health
10	0	0

When I divided my points into an all-or-nothing way, it left me

- *Feeling fat, lazy, and tired all the time because I neglected my health*
- *Sleeping on the couch by myself because I neglected my relationship*
- *Feeling guilty and out of balance by spending too much time in one area*
- *Achieving some "good" results in business, but not "great" ones due to burn out*
- *Unfulfilled*

So... then I tried another way to grow a great, profitable business.

Business	Relationship	Health
6-8	1-2	1-2

This kept me

- *Feeling like I was consistently moving in a great direction*
- *Feeling balanced because I was honoring my focus*
- *Better connected with my relationship and health because I valued the time I had and did not neglect those areas*
- *Achieving "great" results in business and never burning out*
- *Fulfilled*

I determined that if I wanted to grow and be great in any one of my three categories, I must devote six to eight energy points in that one area over a long period of time.

If you desire a great, profitable and fulfilling business, allot your ten energy points like this:

Business	Relationship	Health
6-8	1-2	1-2

If you desire a great, loving and fulfilling relationship, allot your ten energy points like this:

Business	Relationship	Health
1-2	6-8	1-2

If you desire a great, physically able and healthy mind and body, allot your ten energy points like this:

Business	Relationship	Health
1-2	1-2	6-8

The *Why* Behind *How* the Energy Points Are Allotted

Each category requires a daily minimum of one energy point, even if it is not your main focus. For example, in a given day if you do not have any health activities planned, even though there is no conscious, physical energy into your health, it might be in the back of your mind all day. Because of this you might feel some type of guilt associated with neglecting your health. This would do two things:

1) Use up energy that you are not aware of or planned for,
   creating the "energy debt" outlined earlier, and
2) Use up more energy points than necessary.

Remember, your ten energy points consist of physical and emotional energy. If something is on your mind all day, you are "spending" your points!

There's a simple solution! What if you created a conscious choice to honor your decision not to exercise, or not to exercise as much as you wanted that day? If you honor your decision, it will provide clarity and allow you to focus on your business or relationship. By giving yourself permission to only devote one or two energy points to your health that day, those few points go much further. They will especially go further if you have already scheduled other times in your week where you've allotted more energy points to health. This will allow you to relax and become less anxious. Because you are relaxed, you don't consume unnecessary points required for your focus.

Please know that in a given time frame—let's say a week—*all* seven days do not have to be focused on one area. That is extreme, especially if you have many other responsibilities. The guideline for success says that **"most of your points most of the time" are required in one area over a long time frame.** So in a seven-day week, if my focus is business, my energy distribution might look like this:

Chart I	Monday	Tuesday	Wednesday	Thursday	Friday	Saturday	Sunday	Total Energy Points
Business	8	7	8	6	8	1	1	39
Relationship	1	2	1	1	1	7	5	18
Health	1	1	1	3	1	2	4	13
Day Totals	10	10	10	10	10	10	10	70

BEING FULFILLED

It is clear to see from Chart I that during this week most of my energy most of the time was focused on my business, and my daily totals did not go over ten points. To ensure you are creating unlimited wealth, it is important to see that in the Total Energy Points column, other areas of your life are also being honored. Even though your business received most of the points, the other two areas are taken care of and satisfied.

A Note on Energy Points

Your ten energy points might look different than mine or the next person's, meaning that in a similar time frame I might be able to accomplish much more than you can with the same amount of points. Think of energy points being used to do a bicep curl. If you were to do a bicep curl with one of your energy points, maybe right now the most you could curl is twenty pounds. As you train your muscle, it will become stronger and fit. In time you may notice that you can curl forty pounds with that same one energy point.

This is a great example of how over time you can accomplish more with fewer points. Before you trained, in order to curl forty pounds you would have required two energy points. With your new strength gains, it only takes you one! Recognize that everyone is different, and you are only capable of what you are capable of. One thing that is sure to slow you

> down and waste energy points is comparing yourself to others. Focus on your training and on becoming more efficient, and watch each of your energy points become more productive!

"Most of Your Points" – Defined

It is paramount to your success that you understand that "most of your points" mean six to eight points in a given day… no more, no less.

More than Eight Energy Points in One Area:

Notice that in Chart I that I was never a nine or ten in any one category. A nine or ten will signify that you are neglecting other areas completely and not honoring that you are a complete person with other needs. If you focus more than eight points in one area for too long, you'll begin to neglect other areas and will increase your risk of going into energy debt, as expressed earlier. Not only will you increase your odds of burnout, but you will also be unable to create unlimited wealth, because you will become unfulfilled in the area or areas you are neglecting.

Less than Six Energy Points in Your Focus Area:

Having less than six energy points focused in your main area will not produce a great enough result. Look at the figure below.

Business	Relationship	Health
5	2	3

Even though this energy point distribution makes my business *look* like my focus, it is not my *main* focus. The only way you will begin to achieve *significant* results in one area is when you begin to consistently invest six to eight points. Less than six energy points will do a good job of maintaining an area and keeping it average... but in order to grow and be great, six to eight points is required.

"Most of Your Time" – Defined

"Most of Your Time" Each Week:

Most of your time each week means five to six days. It is imperative that you understand that magnificent results don't come on a part-time basis. Less than five days of major focus in any one area just does not produce significant growth over time, especially if you are in your first six years of growing a business or improving your health.

"Most of Your Time" Each Day:

In a given day, determine how many waking hours you have. If you are up at 6:30 a.m. and go to sleep at 10:30 p.m., that's a sixteen-hour day. Given that scenario, "most of your time" would be defined as nine to eleven hours. This can be defined as full time. Take a look at Chart II.

Chart II	*Day 1*
Business	8
Relationship	1
Health	1

According to Chart II, day one might look like this for me: Wake up at 6:30 a.m. and be with my son until 9:00 a.m. Work my business from

9:00 a.m. until 5:00 p.m. From 5:00 pm till 7:30 p.m., be with my family, go for a walk together and eat healthy. From 7:30 p.m. to 8:30 p.m., be with my wife. From 8:30 p.m. until 10:30 p.m., work on my business. That is ten hours on my business, two-and-a-half with my son, two-and-a-half with my family and an hour with my wife. In this case, I am honoring all three areas of my life with a major focus on business.

I have created the situation where I work from home so I can literally be with my son until 8:59 a.m., perform my thirty-second commute upstairs to my office and be ready for 9:00 a.m.. I realize that your situation may be different with commuting time, having a job, and a side business, having many children, social events after and or before work, etc. I bet your list goes on and on. The whole point of this new model for fulfillment is to understand that you cannot have all those things in your day and create unlimited wealth... you must take as many activities out of your day as possible to succeed. Notice in the example above, I am a businessman and family man... that is all!

How to Get Rid of Many Areas and Feel Okay

To attain my fulfillment in business, I have weeded out things that use my valuable energy points—things like commute time, unnecessary networking, meetings, jobs, volunteering my time, hobbies, the time I spend with friends and family, certain exercise times, unnecessary phone calls, and internet time. I had to set my boundaries and get to the point with people. I began to invest my time wisely and produce in the time I had versus the time I wished for. I created big sacrifices to attain significant fulfillment.

BEING FULFILLED

While I removed a lot of energy point consumers, what I did not do is neglect the important areas. Because my focus was business, I had to ask to myself, "What must I absolutely have in my other two categories of relationships and health?" My answers were: my son, my wife, friends and family contact, and exercise time. I weeded out *everything* else! Outside of my major business focus, I scheduled a couple exercise times a week, had a few hours each day for my wife and son, and contacted my friends and family on a very limited basis. I became clear on what items would serve my vision and which ones would detract from my vision. Anything that pulled me away, I did not even look at.

Once you determine what boundaries are necessary, communication with others and yourself are the key. Talk to your spouse, your friends, and your family about what you are looking to do. Be as direct and clear as possible with what you require from them and what you are looking to do. Communicate with yourself about what is necessary or not. You deserve to get honest with yourself for this process to work.

This communication with all necessary parties essentially gives you permission to focus most of your points most of the time on one area. If you have any guilt driven by yourself or inflicted by others, you will burn up unnecessary and valuable energy points, and you will know that you have not communicated effectively.

As you progress with this process, the key to your fulfillment is to **become great at producing bigger results from one point that you currently do from ten.** This is accomplished by practicing the habit of focus.

About Focus

Think of focus as priority mail. Priority mail gets there in the least amount of time because the postal service promises to "focus" their energy to get your package there quickly. Priority mail costs more than regular mail because it takes more energy to get the job done faster. Realize that regular mail still gets to the destination; it just takes more time.

In the case of humans, when we have a priority focus, things get done more quickly and the effort it takes seems less. When we are not focused on one area, we can still arrive at a desired result; however, the odds of us getting there are greatly decreased. People get distracted, people lose ambition, people forget, and people are above all… human. It's been said, "To err is human." Exactly! That is why focus is imperative. When you have focus, you are less likely to err. If you do err, then it will not slow you down, because you are focused.

Focus keeps your attention on what you are doing. Lack of focus keeps your attention on what you are not doing. Focus is fuel. Focus creates more time because you can accomplish more in less time. Focus releases stress because tasks do not require as much effort to do them. Stress is caused from thinking too much. Focus shuts the brain down and allows you to operate from the heart… from a place called trust.

Let's look at some facts to see what we have established so far with this new model for fulfillment:

- *Each of the three categories clearly depends on the others.*
- *In order to be truly great in any category, we must have consistent laser focus with repetitive, productive action over a long period of time... in ONE AREA.*
- *While focusing on that one area, we must feel like we are not neglecting the other two.*
- *We can only be great in one area at any one time.*
- *We are limited to the energy we have each day and no more (Ten Points).*
- *If you use more than ten energy points, you will burn out quickly.*
- *In order to succeed you must invest most of your points most of the time in one area.*
- *We must become great at producing bigger results from one point than we currently do from ten.*
- *We can produce bigger results from fewer points by setting up boundaries with others and ourselves via great, clear communication.*

The Big Picture

To achieve unlimited wealth, you must understand that it is a process that does take some time. It requires you to be patient and to understand where you are in your life at any one point. During this process, ask lots of questions to help yourself understand what you want, what your responsibilities are, how what you "want" fits into those responsibilities, and most importantly, where your focus is most appropriate.

Bigger than all that would be to understand *how to achieve what you want without sacrificing other important areas*. Because if you can achieve greatness in an area without feeling like you are sacrificing the others, fulfillment is soon to follow. This is a huge component of this model, and it's the key to your fulfillment. Even though the other areas are not necessarily improving, they are not being ignored or neglected.

Let's be clear and recognize that life can get in the way of even the strongest focus by a death in the family, a health problem, a real need for money, quitting your job, divorce, the birth of a child, or a family crisis. With this in mind, ask yourself: "Where is most of my energy and most of my time appropriate at this given point in my life?" If you want to focus on your business but your spouse wants a divorce, if you care at all about the relationship, you'd better put your business on maintenance mode, or at least have a serious conversation.

Most people run into the problem of temporarily fixing something and thinking everything is fine.

Health Example:
    If you went to the doctor and found out you have high blood pressure and high cholesterol, you'd better shift your focus to your health for a while to get it under control. What most people do is go on medication to lower their blood pressure and cholesterol versus carving out time for a regular

exercise and healthier eating program. Medication is a temporary fix and does not solve anything.

Relationship Example:

I have coached clients who were in rocky relationships. They wanted a more fulfilling relationship, but their focus was clearly somewhere else. Their attitude, like many others, was to try and fix everything in one date or one conversation. I would ask them: "How often do you and your spouse communicate on real issues outside of the children, work, or your day?" The bottom line answer was that most couples only truly communicate when there is something wrong. They get upset, have an argument, get angry for a period of time, have a great, heartfelt conversation, sometimes have make-up sex, and go right back to doing what brought them to the initial argument until it boils over again.

In both of these examples, to create true, sustained changes requires most of their energy points most of the time over a long period of time. If they do not shift their focus to the appropriate category, the result is as good as a plumber coming to your house to fix a leaky pipe and sticking chewing gum in the crack.

The big picture of this model to attain unlimited wealth recognizes life's unique changes. By understanding where most of your energy and time is required at a particular phase in your life, you are better able to remain stress free and produce great results. **The big picture is to be so focused in one area for a long enough time so that when you shift your focus onto another area, the initial area does not suffer because it is in such great condition.**

Example

A client, Ron, has a passion for fitness and health, and this is where he has invested most of his energy and most of his time over a twenty-year period. Because he started young and kicked his unhealthy habits early enough, Ron created a very high level of physical and mental health. Several years ago, when it was time to get serious about growing his business, he recognized that if he wanted serious results, he deserved to take some time away from his health-related activities. Essentially he shifted his six to eight points to his business.

Because he had created a high level of health over the past twenty years, he could maintain great health with only three workouts each week versus his usual eight. By removing five workouts each week, he could allot the majority of his energy points to his business. In doing this, after only three years of truly focusing on his business, Ron created some incredible results. They weren't the type of results at this point where he could shift his focus and expect to maintain them like he was able to maintain his health, but they were very impressive. He recognized that with another solid chunk of time, he would absolutely be in a position where he could once again shift his main focus if necessary.

In the meantime, while focusing on his business, Ron was continually assessing his relationship and his health. During this time, he had consistent communication with his wife to ensure they were on the same page with each of their focuses. Remember, communication is essential. While there might be periods of time where Ron's major focus will shift a little, this must be appropriate and communicated.

Take a look at some real life emails I have collected from my most fulfilled clients over the years who have applied this new model for fulfillment. Notice how these people are recognizing, honoring, and communicating where their focus is appropriate.

> *Dear Jeff,*
> *I am thrilled to talk to my friend for you. Please know that he has made himself very unavailable because there have been some family issues in his life, and I know that he is focusing much more on his family lately and not much else.*

> *Dear Jeff,*
> *I would love to write you a testimonial, but it will have to be at the end of the summer. I have some great opportunities in my business and all of my focus is being directed there.*

> *Dear Jeff,*
> *I am writing to let you know that I would like to postpone my business focus for a while. I have been so focused on my business lately that my relationship has gone down the toilet. I am pulling away from many areas of my life so that I can utilize most of my energy to improve my relationship.*

Dear Jeff,

My brother-in-law suffered a massive heart attack and is now on life support and will probably die within a few days. I am doing the minimum that I can with all aspects of my life and focusing on him and my family.

Dear Jeff,

I would like the focus of our coaching to be on my health. Over the past twenty years I have built a multimillion dollar organization, but I have let my health suffer in the process. My main focus over the next several years is to drastically improve my health!

Dear Jeff,

I cannot believe that my daughter is going to college. I feel so guilty, because for her complete childhood I was so focused on my business. I feel like I have missed out. I don't regret building my business; I just wish I had devoted a bit more time to her on a weekly basis.

Dear Jeff,

I have been implementing our discussions from our coaching sessions by communicating better with my husband. It is amazing how supportive he is! Now I can put the majority of my focus on my health and not feel like my relationship is melting away.

BEING FULFILLED

Dear Jeff,

Remember when we first began coaching I wanted a better relationship with my wife, but it seemed like I never had the time to focus on her because I was so focused with my business? I know that sounded bad, but I felt I couldn't leave my business without it folding. I have been sharing with her how I feel, and as a result, we have scheduled a date night once a week. After three months of sticking to this, it is amazing how much closer and satisfied we both are! She recognizes that I must focus on the business, and it turns out that all we both required was knowing that we would spend some quality time together each week.

SECTION II

THE CORE STAGES AND PHILOSOPHIES

The Seven Stages
to Achieving Unlimited Wealth

In the first section I presented you with a simple model consisting of three categories: Business, Relationships, and Health. Since almost everyone is seeking unlimited wealth (complete fulfillment) in these areas and having little sustained success, I stressed that to attain this wealth our efforts must be focused on one area for a long time. Recognizing that you only have so much energy each day (ten points) it is imperative that you determine which of the three categories is appropriate for you to focus on. Once you determine which category requires your focus, you can begin to apply a seven-stage process in that category to assist you with your fulfillment.

These stages can be applied to each of the three categories that comprise unlimited wealth, but *only one at a time*. The following section is a brief overview of the seven stages and the ten key philosophies to assist you in their implementation. The remainder of the book will apply the seven stages specifically in each of the three categories.

BEING FULFILLED

The Seven Stages to Achieve Unlimited Wealth

Stage 1: *Create a Vision*

Stage 2: *Simplify and Prioritize from that Vision*

Stage 3: *Structure and Organize Your Days around Your Priorities*

Stage 4: *Know Yourself and Establish Your New Rules*

Stage 5: *Find the Right People to Maintain the Focus and Support Your Vision*

Stage 6: *Maintain Focus on that Vision and from that Vision*

Stage 7: *Practice and Duplication*

Stage 1:
Create a Vision

What is your definition of "vision?" Take a moment to write your definition on the lines below.

Vision is:_____

_____

_____

There is no right or wrong answer to this question. Vision is exactly how you see it. Walt Disney said, "If you can dream it, you can do it." This sums up the power of creating a vision. Realize that vision is foresight, imagination, mental images, a revelation, visualization, dreams, ideas, prediction, and so much more.

The only way you will create massive results in any of the three categories is to create a vision that is clear and certain. Without this clarity and certainty, you will be simply floating in a dream. You will use phrases like, "I hope to someday…" or "Maybe I will…" or "I wish I could…" You will know when your vision is clear when you have an overwhelming urge to move forward, when every cell in your body is in alignment with this vision. If so much as one cell disagrees, you will experience resistance and be less likely to succeed.

> Think of a clear and certain vision as a court trial. The "jury" represents the cells in your body. Your vision must convince every member of the "jury" beyond a reasonable doubt that this vision is the right one and that it deserves all of your focus long-term. If so much as one "juror," or cell, does not agree, the vision is dismissed.

What is the purpose of a vision? Take a moment to write your definition on the lines below.

The purpose of a vision is: _____

_____

_____

Once you have seen the path through your clear and certain vision, your fulfillment is no longer a matter of "if" it will happen but a matter of "when" it will happen. The certainty that your vision provides allows you to no longer even care about the "when," because you are 100% sure that it will happen, and this allows you to focus on the immediate action to bring your vision into fruition.

Example: When you *know* you will become a millionaire, from a clear and certain vision, the focus on and need to become one right now goes away. You now have the ability to focus on the tasks at hand versus worrying and stressing. This focused manner allows you to produce bigger results more quickly and with less effort. A clear and certain vision gets rid of all the fear, doubt, anxiety, and overwhelmed feelings. **A vision grounds you so that you can take purposeful steps in an intelligent direction.** Without a vision, there is nothing to focus on, and you will feel like you are floating in the middle of the ocean with no sight of land.

Stage 2:
Simplify and Prioritize from that Vision

When your vision is clear and certain enough, you will quickly realize that many of the "to-dos" in your life are very inappropriate for your given focus. The difficult part of this is that these inappropriate to-dos are more often than not things you really want to do in your life. These can consist of hobbies, television shows, people, and sports. Take a look again at Figure D. This is the stage where you begin to get the red ink out and cross things off!

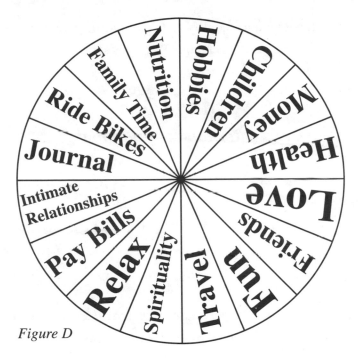

Figure D

It is imperative that you simplify your life to as few things as possible by effective communication. Remember that you have only ten precious energy points to distribute each day. As you know from experience, these go very quickly. You do not have to like this simplification process... liking is not required. There will be many things you do not like but know intuitively and logically they make sense. Besides, if the vision is truly powerful, simplifying your life should be that much easier.

Once you have simplified your life, it is time to prioritize the activities and commitments you have left. I am sure you have heard of prioritizing before; however, here is used with real power. There are certain levels of priority... high, medium, and low. You must recognize at which level priority your actions are before you can recognize if you are the best person to be doing them. If low-priority items can be done by other people or cut out completely, your ten energy points will go further.

If you find it hard to simplify and then prioritize, odds are that your vision is not clear and certain enough. Revisit Stage 1.

Stage 3:

Structure and Organize Your Days around Your Priorities

Your vision will provide many clues as to what actions will be required from you on a daily basis. We all know that without action, a vision remains only a vision. If you are having any trouble creating action, three things are possible.

1) Your vision is not clear and certain enough. Revisit Stage 1.

2) You have not simplified your life enough. Revisit Stage 2

3) Your days are not structured enough, and you are disorganized.

This stage is appropriate when number three is your situation. This is the time to create a structure of when and where your ten points are to be used. What is your schedule like? What is the first thing you will do when you wake up? When do you go to bed? What systems are you using to produce the most from each energy point you use? How organized are you? **If any of these questions bring up an uneasy feeling, this stage is even more important for you!**

Beyond having a vision, the majority of people are not fulfilled because they are not organized and have no regular structure to their day. Know that just having a clear vision does not mean you will automatically achieve fulfillment. This stage will not only teach you how to become organized and structured, but it will teach you the value of it as well. The main objective here is to take the priorities you discovered from Stage Two and structure them into your day with uncompromisable time.

Uncompromisable time is time you have set aside in your schedule week to week that no matter what, you honor. If getting to the gym on Mondays at 4:30 p.m. is a high priority and you've blocked it out in your schedule as uncompromisable time, a networking meeting or anything else cannot replace it under any circumstances (besides obvious tragedies). *Uncompromisable time for activities outside your main focus area will ensure that you don't neglect those areas.*

With your newfound structure and organization you will be able to easily find a place to fit in all your priorities from Stage Two. Once you determine those priorities, it is imperative that you fit them into your structured day. This is why you must simplify so much in Stage Two. You will soon realize that no matter how organized and structured you are, there are many priorities that require your attention in one area. Coming to terms with simplicity and structure is imperative, because a lack of structure and the guilty emotions around it will zap your energy points. Here are a couple funny quotes I have heard from coaching clients of mine:

**"The lack of structure makes it harder for
me to enjoy the lack of structure."**
- A retired client

"I am feeling guilty about feeling guilty."
- Client

Stage 4:
Know Yourself and Establish Your New Rules

In order to attain unlimited wealth at this stage, understanding yourself is paramount. Now that you have created a vision in your focus area, simplified and prioritized your life, and created the structure and organization to put it into... *it is necessary to understand how you perform in this new environment.* How well do you handle stressful situations? How do you react under certain emotions... fear, overwhelm, guilt, chaos, frustration, or confusion? What situations can you create to maximize your performance? What circumstances occur that drain unnecessary energy points?

This stage is dedicated to attaining a better understanding of your internal and external environment. This stage has a simple process:

1) Create an Awareness of Current Behaviors
2) Identify Triggers and Current Rules
3) Consciously Practice New Responses

Here you create an awareness of what keeps you doing the same thing over and over again. You identify the triggers and rules that set your old behavior patterns in motion, and then you break those old patterns by practicing new responses and creating a new rule book. Essentially, you will learn to create rules that serve you versus those that hold you back, and begin to challenge everything you know to see how it fits into your new focus. You will learn from past mistakes by studying both your successes and failures. You will understand what to duplicate and what not to duplicate. When you understand yourself, you attain better results.

Stage 5:
Find the Right People to Maintain the Focus and Support Your Vision

My great friend and author, Lois Tiedemann, wrote a book I highly recommend called *No One Succeeds Alone*. She is right! Stage Five is not just about finding people, it is about finding the right people. Without a support network, mentor network, coaching network, training network, and personal network, your long-term fulfillment just is not possible. Think of a time when you tried something by yourself... a time when you refused to ask for help. How long did it take to do it on your own? How much quicker would it have been if you had a team assisting you?

Because we as individuals only have ten energy points each day, **we must find a way to leverage other people's ten points toward our results.** You've already learned that in order to maintain the focus on your vision, you must eliminate as much as possible from Stage Two. Once this is done, you want to find the right people to do as much for you as possible so you can focus your ten points on activities that produce results.

You cannot hire someone to run on the treadmill for you, but you can hire someone to go grocery shopping for you. You cannot hire someone to spend some quality time with your spouse, but you can hire someone to do the bookkeeping for your business. **Leveraging other people's energy points to produce bigger results in your life is another key to creating unlimited wealth.**

Stage 6:

*Maintain Focus **on that** Vision and **from that** Vision*

With each day that passes, your every cell is focused on that original vision. Your every thought seems to revert back to this vision. Maintaining focus on that vision should be easy because the vision is so clear. Think of your vision as a vacuum. This vacuum creates a giant tunnel and sucks you in. This tunnel provides extreme focus and automatically sets boundaries for you. It blocks out all the objects that you previously stumbled upon, all the people that sucked your time, and all the tasks that depleted your energy.

When you are in this tunnel, it is easy to say no to people because your direction is so clear. It is easy to see if opportunities that come your way distract you from your vision or allow you to get there quicker. There will, however, be days where life gets in the way. This is where you will use this stage to maintain focus on your vision. If your vision is clear and certain enough, maintaining focus will be easy, and taking the necessary time away from this vision to deal with life will not feel distracting. In fact, no matter how bad the circumstances are, if your vision is powerful enough, you will always find opportunities in your day's away from the vision to assist your overall results.

If you find it hard to maintain focus on your vision, revisit Stage 1. Continue through each stage again to ensure you have done everything possible to streamline your life and focus your energy points appropriately.

Stage 7:
Practice and Duplication

The power of practice and repetition! This is fundamental and simple yet not acted upon enough. With everything you have done to this point, Stage Seven is where great habits are formed. While the value of practice and repetition may be clear logically for you, until you *experience the results* of that practice, it might be more difficult for you to maintain ongoing action. This difficulty is due to the lack of habit. This stage is ironic, because the main objective of Stage Seven is to form great habits via practice, yet the very lack of a great habit might make it more difficult to begin or keep going.

This is why all the other stages come before this one. Your clear vision, your simple life, your strong structure, and your knowledge of yourself and the right people will be your fuel when times get tough. Once you begin to practice all of the previous stages, your new habits are more likely to be formed.

> The free throw is a fundamental of basketball. For those of you unfamiliar with basketball, when an offensive player is taking a shot and the defense makes unreasonable contact to distract the shot, it's called a foul. The offensive player then has an opportunity to take two "free" shots fifteen feet from the basket with no defense to get in the way. Free throws are always taken from the same place on the court. How important are free throws in basketball? Games are won and lost on free throws. If you took every close game in the history of basketball and looked at

how many free throws the losing team missed, I bet if the losing team had made even half of their missed free throws, they would have won that game.

John Wooden was a college basketball coach known most for teaching fundamentals. His teams won eleven consecutive national championships, unlike any team in history. His teams won seven in a row, whereas the next closest team won only three in a row. How did he do this? Sure he coached some superstars, but the majority of his teams consisted of "average" athletes. His success rested on repetition and practice of fundamentals.

He would take an athlete, the best or the worst, and make them shoot four hundred free throws every practice. He knew that games were won or lost on the fundamentals, and he knew the habits of a championship team. When you are in a game, any game, and there is no time left on the clock, your team is down by one, and you are at the free throw line with two shots, what do you want to rely on—habits or luck? When an "average" athlete is under pressure, they choke or pass the ball. When a "superstar" athlete is under pressure, habit kicks in and the victory is effortless and thrilling.

While you are practicing, you must be keenly aware of how you can duplicate what you are doing and have done... especially when you succeed. Most people that struggle today have had some success in their lives. Their problem is not that they cannot succeed again, but rather that they cannot duplicate their previous successes. **You must be able to duplicate your success by leaving a trail you can follow back any time you want.**

If you are walking for miles in the woods and suddenly come across a beautiful waterfall, how would you find it again? The easiest way would be to leave a trail. Fulfillment is no different. When you achieve great victories or are in fantastic moods, how do you duplicate this? Success leaves clues; it is up to you to become aware of those clues by leaving a trail.

After your victory party, sit down and ask yourself some thought-provoking questions. Discover what you did and the path you chose to arrive at your success. Record this valuable information so you can duplicate your success again and again with half the effort.

Ten Key Philosophies
for Your Fulfillment

Your fulfillment in life is stapled to your philosophy. There is no other way around this fact. When you change your philosophy, you change your results. As a personal trainer and success coach for thousands of people, I have come to understand human behavior at a very deep level. This section focuses all that knowledge, expertise, and personal experience into ten key philosophies. These philosophies are necessary to understand before you begin to apply the seven stages to an area of your life, because they provide a foundation on which to build your results. Adopting these key philosophies will allow you to become fulfilled sooner.

Philosophy #1:
Embrace and Understand Change

For all you out there who hate change… I am sure there is a club to join. There are people that embrace change; however, if you are not one of them, I suggest you take a moment to understand that change is a key element in your immediate and long-term fulfillment. No matter who you are, it is important to understand what change is and what it means to you. Let's begin by asking: How would you define change? Write your answer in the space below.

Change is _____

_____

What does change mean to you?

Change means _____

_____

Is your overall definition of change and the meaning of it more negative or positive? Many people hate change for three reasons:

1) They do not understand it.

2) They don't think they are good at it.

3) They have a negative association when they think of it.

Most of the time it's not change that you don't like, it's the feeling inside that you have lost control. Have you ever been happy with the way life was going, and then something changed? This meant you *had to* do something different when you really did not *want to*. Most people struggle with the fact that change is about control. Who has control… you or the event?

It's important to realize that we have complete control over our internal environment but very little, if any, over our external environment. That being said, when an external event happens, like someone smashing the windows in your car, you can feel like you have lost control. The fact is that you really don't have control over that event, whether you like it or not. Your windows are smashed. What you do have control over is your response to the event.

BEING FULFILLED

Though it may not seem like it, you always have complete control over your thoughts and responses. Fulfillment is a choice. Your results are choices. In the case of your trashed car, you have two choices: 1) You can choose to react negatively, point fingers, and blame others, or 2) You can choose to respond by asking, "How am I going to resolve this situation?" While this is not always easy to do, you must remember the bottom line: change is a struggle between who has the power. When you let go of what you cannot control and focus on what you can, you are in your power!

Most people think that in order to change they must begin by changing. Those are the people that never get started, because you can't just "change." When you say that you want to change, very often, the focus is on what you want to change; i.e., the bad habit, the negative thought, or the failed result. Remember that what you focus on grows. If you are focusing on changing what you don't want, all your energy is wrapped around the disempowering item. So how *do* we change? Let's break it down into three stages—think of it as **CPR**:

> *1) The **C**reation… Here you say: "I am creating something new."*
> *2) The **P**rocess… Here you say: "I am changing."*
> *3) The **R**esult… Here you say: "I have changed."*

1) The Creation: To begin the process of change you must create something new. Have you ever said, "I have to change this negative thought into a positive one," or "I have to change this bad habit into a good one?" Very few of us succeed in changing something bad into something good. Here's why. Let's pretend a bad event is an apple and a good event is an orange. When you say, "I have to change this bad event into a good one," essentially you are trying to change an apple into an orange. Okay,

Houdini… And you wonder why you have struggled so much. You cannot change an apple into an orange. An apple is an apple, and a bad event is a bad event.

While you cannot change a bad event into good one, you can create a new perspective about an event. Most people struggle to change without seeing any results because they are trying to change the event, not creating a new perspective about the event. **Fulfillment comes when you create something new versus trying to change something old.** In this first stage of change, you begin by creating a new perspective, belief, thought, emotion, situation, or dream. This new vision literally pulls your focus away from what you don't want and wraps it around your new, empowering vision. Here you say: *"I am creating something new."*

2) The Process: Once you have created your new belief, thought, etc., you can begin the process of change. This is where all the action takes place. As you practice these new beliefs and thoughts, you will notice new behaviors. You are now changing. This stage is dynamic. When you practice these new thoughts long enough, they begin to become subconscious actions that don't take much energy to perform. The process is where you develop new habits. Here you say: *"I am changing."*

3) The Result: As these new habits kick in, you will begin to see new results in your life. Essentially you have become someone different to attain a new result. You are now changed. Here you say: *"I have changed."*

Philosophy #2:
Great Habits Produce Great Results

How to Create a Habit

We are embarking on a philosophy that is one of the most valuable components of fulfillment: habits... great habits! Your fulfillment in business, relationships, and health lies in the habits you possess. These three categories are connected via similar habits. *This philosophy is about how to create those habits and the barriers that might get in your way.*

Your current habits produce the current results you experience right now. Compare a person with the habit of brushing and flossing his or her teeth every morning and evening to the person who does that only occasionally. Whose teeth are in better shape? I know you get it, but do you really? This experience is not about pointing out the obvious, but rather diving deep inside a habit to understand how to form one.

Habits are just as simple as a man's mind. Jerry Seinfeld said, "Do you really want to know what men are thinking? Nothing... men are just wandering around thinking about nothing." (Some of you woman may disagree!) Habits are not complicated; they just are repetitive, subconscious, and they produce a result. Let's keep it simple: a bad habit produces a bad result. A great habit produces a great result.

One day of a great habit produces one great feeling that leads to one great result. What about three months of a great habit—or a year, two years, ten years? My client Joe had adopted the great habit of lifting weights at a high intensity three times a week since 1994. To date, that is thirteen years. What result do you think *that* thirteen-year habit has produced for Joe… a beer belly or a six-pack?

Habits are formed from many feelings that we experience over and over again. **Feelings produce habits, and habits produce results.** As humans, when we experience something over and over again (like a feeling), it becomes familiar and we begin to like it. It becomes part of the family, so to speak. That feeling can be good or bad for us; either way, we are familiar with it, and therefore we like it.

"Hooked on a Feeling"

There is a line from a song that says *"...hooked on a feeling."* That is exactly what we do. Have you ever been in love? It does not matter if that person is good or bad for you; in the beginning when everything is rosy, all you experience is love. When you experience that love feeling frequently enough, you get "hooked" on it.

If a couple is truly not a good match, often those feelings they became hooked on in the beginning of a relationship can cloud their judgment even when they are gone. The addiction to wanting that feeling again can allow someone to stay in a bad relationship for years. Even though the "love" may be gone, the feelings around the relationship become familiar and comfortable.

Because habits are formed from feelings, it's important to understand that a **habit is a feeling we crave to experience on a daily basis.** Your habit says: *I crave to feel a certain way; do whatever is necessary to feel it*. Remember Joe's habit of lifting weights? He was not hooked on lifting weights; he was hooked on how he felt before, during, and after he lifted them. He craved feeling that way, so he did the action necessary to produce that feeling. Over time, Joe did it so much that he formed a habit. Doing something consistently over time is what trains the body to become familiar with it, and this creates a lasting habit. That familiarity creates routine, so the action becomes subconscious. This subconscious part of habits is a vital component as to why they work.

The Sugar High

Have you ever been motivated? I mean *really* motivated. Maybe you read a book, saw a movie, attended a seminar, hired a coach, or had a conversation with someone. I know you have been there… all fired up and motivated, ready to revolutionize your life. You saw it so clearly, and you vowed to yourself and others that things would change. You said things like, "It's done," "I can do it!" and "Finally my time has come." When you got home, you threw away old things, cleaned out closets, joined a gym, had a family meeting, went for a five-mile jog, or wrote in your journal all night.

You were good for a few days or so… at best for a couple of weeks. With a blink of an eye, before you knew it, six months had passed and you found that expired gym membership or that old journal you passionately wrote in. Somehow you had reverted back to the way you were before that motivating experience. You say to yourself, "But I was so sure"; "I really thought this time was it"; "I thought I was ready." If you are like most people, you begin to blame yourself. What really happened?

2:00 a.m. Motivation

Picture it... it is two a.m., and you are fighting to keep your eyes open. You are sitting in front of the television with an empty bag of chips, a bottle of wine, *and* a bowl of ice cream! You suddenly are awakened by a loud infomercial with this hot chick and a buffed out guy wearing next to nothing doing abdominal crunches with this odd looking device on a beach in California.

The voice from the television says: "You too can have abs like this in only minutes a day!" There you are three minutes later on the phone with your credit card, making three easy payments of $19.95. After you place the order, you are "motivated." You are so proud of yourself. You are thinking that once this machine comes in two to three weeks, you are going to change everything. So, to celebrate this newfound success, you break open a new bag of cookies and munch on them guiltlessly—because you are on the path to success!

BEING FULFILLED

> We have all had these moments in our own way. This motivation dupes us into believing, even for a moment, that we can change a thirty-year sedentary habit in a moment's rush. The fact is, motivation cannot change a habit; it cannot change thirty years of sitting on the couch every night. All the excitement in the world cannot change what is so subconsciously routine and normal to you.

The bottom line is that motivation is like a sugar high; it will leave you tired and craving more. What most people don't take into consideration is what they have been doing for the previous thirty years before that motivational experience. **Great habits are the key to fulfillment because when the initial excitement or motivation of an experience wears off, habits kick in.** If you allow old habits to kick in, they will produce old, familiar results.

Motivation is important to begin a process; however, is it only a catalyst to start. It is up to you to recognize when that catalyst wears off and what behaviors you tend to revert back to. So how do we change old habits into better ones?

Remember the three stages from Philosophy #1, C.P.R. In order to kick an old habit, you simply stop using it by creating a new one, leaving the old one to rust. It's that simple! Example: Pick something you are good at that requires frequent practice. Maybe it is a sport, a hobby, or a special skill you have. Stop doing it for twenty years, and then pick it up again. How difficult would it be to be great at it after twenty years of not doing it? This is perfect proof that when you don't practice something, it deteriorates. When you focus on the new habit and practice it day by day, you improve. It may not be easy, but things in life that are truly rewarding are never easy.

Potential Barriers

Has anyone ever broken off a relationship with you and said, "It's not you... It's me." People hear that line and for some reason blame themselves, even though the other person said, "It was not you!" Most people think it was something they said or did or even something they did not do that caused the breakup. They begin to think it *was* them! This is called the *It's my fault syndrome*.

One of the behaviors that will get in your way of creating a new habit is blaming yourself for the old ones. If you truly want to succeed in creating unlimited wealth, it is important for you to separate yourself from your habits. You and your habits are two separate entities. A habit is a learned behavior based on your environment and past experiences. Who you are as a person and the values you possess on the inside have nothing to do with your habits.

You can value your health dearly, yet still be a chain-smoker. The smoking does not define you, the value does. Most people will allow a habit to define who they are. The difficult part of this comes when they want to kick a bad habit, because they feel they have to change who they are inside which can be very difficult. When creating a new habit, you will be a different person in your mindset, but you don't have to change who you are. Let's keep this simple: **Create a new habit, not a new you.** Your values—not your habits—define who you are.

If you are looking to create new habits, realize that nothing is wrong with you. You do not have to fix you; it is not your fault. It's not you... it's the habit! I hope this releases some pressure for you. Many of my clients in the process of change have had difficulty because they held themselves responsible for all their poor habits and kept blaming themselves. When they recognized that it was not their fault, everything changed. They stopped allowing their habits to define who they were and began to define themselves through their values. This is the foundation of my coaching called "The True You," where you discover your authentic self and who you truly are. Realize that poor habits are just that—poor habits... *they are not you!*

Four Steps to a New Habit

Step One: *Identify the habit that does not serve you, drop it, and create a new one*

Step Two: *Consciously practice the new habit you wish to adopt*

Step Three: *Educate your expectations*

Step Four: *Go back through Steps Two and Three*

Envision your habits, good or bad, as a shirt you can take off. It is that simple. **Step one in creating a new habit is to identify the one that does not serve you, drop it, and create a new one.** Once you identify it, take it off. You can do this step by asking:

- *What habits do I currently express which produce my present result?*
- *What are the habits of a person who has what I want?*
- *Which of these new habits would serve me better?*

Once you identify these, the learning process begins. Habits are learned and practiced... consciously or subconsciously. Because the habits that do not serve you were most likely learned subconsciously, you can learn a new one, but it must be consciously. **Step two in creating a new habit is consciously practicing the new habit you wish to adopt.** If you want to learn to play tennis, you pick up a racquet and play. You may hire a coach and require partners, but at the end of the day, if you want to get better, you must play.

If you want to create a new habit, you must practice it. A perfect example would be to look at how long you have been practicing the habits you wish to release. The only reason they seem so hard to let go of is because you have been practicing them for so long. If you have overeaten for twenty years and are twenty pounds overweight, it would seem reasonable and even logical that it might possibly take twenty years to reverse that habit of overeating and releasing that weight. So why do people get upset when they work out for three months and have not yet lost the twenty pounds?

In order to prevent this frustration, we use **Step Three in creating a new habit: Educate your expectations.** Please stop lying to yourself and pretending not to know what you know. An unmet expectation always leads to disappointment. If your friend began a workout program looking to release one hundred pounds and came to you three weeks later saying, "I'm going to quit. I have worked my butt off for three weeks, and I have only lost five pounds," what would you say to them?

If they invested five to ten years of working hard every day, *really* following the guidelines and playing by the rules, then they might have some ground to stand on. The fact is, you know what it takes for fulfillment, but most people are unwilling to put that type of effort in. Most will pretend not to know what they know and begin to expect failure. When you educate your expectations and get honest, you will achieve with ease.

Step Four in creating a new habit is going back through Steps Two and Three. Practice, educate… practice, educate! You begin to practice your new habit, and when you become stuck or frustrated, you look at your expectation and educate it. This is the time to get honest, take the pressure off, and get back to the practice part.

Philosophy Summary

It is important to tie together what we have discussed to maximize your results. So far, I've showed you how feelings form habits. Those feelings you experience on a regular basis are responsible for the habits you form. Your habits drive your daily actions. Because of the repetition necessary to produce a habit, you become very familiar with those actions, and they become very subconscious. When we want to begin the process of change in our lives, habits are the key to success because when the initial excitement or motivation of an experience wears off, habits kick in. If you rely on your old habits, you will see old results. In order to successfully go through the process of change, you begin by creating something new. Fulfillment comes when you create a new habit versus trying to change an old one. Don't change an old habit; create a new one and the other will rust from neglect. Like playing a sport, if you quit, you naturally lose the skill.

A major role in your fulfillment stems from the acceptance that you are not at fault for the bad habits that you may have. Habits are simply learned from your environment and past experiences, and they do not define who you are. The process of forming a new habit seems a bit simpler when you only have to create a new habit and not a new you. In order to begin this process, remember the four steps in creating a new habit:

Step One: *Identify the habit that does not serve you, drop it, and create a new one*

Step Two: *Consciously practice the new habit you wish to adopt*

Step Three: *Educate your expectations*

Step Four: *Go back through Steps Two and Three*

Never forget that your habits will produce your results. So if you want better results, it is as simple as creating a better habit using these four steps and mastering this information.

Coach's Challenge

Of all the information presented so far, practice and repetition is the most important factor in adopting a new habit. Just like in sports: a truly great athlete has mastered his game in practice. As a professional athlete, you get paid on how well you perform in clutch moments. Every professional athlete is excellent; that is why they are professionals. What separates an "average" professional athlete from a "superstar" is not natural ability but practice and repetition.

What habits are necessary for you to become a championship leader? What habits are necessary for you to create unlimited wealth? Are you relying on habits or luck to determine your fulfillment? The goal is for you to master a new habit. When people say, "Teach me something new," I know they are not into mastery. If you are a master of none, then you will have nothing! If you want to master anything, you must do it over and over again.

How many times will you have to take the shot before you master it? As many as it requires for the desired result. If you are seeking ten new sales a month, how many people are you required to meet with? As many as it requires to achieve ten sales. If you are seeking to release ten pounds over the next three months, how many workouts are necessary? As many as it requires to release the ten pounds.

The Challenge

Pick an activity in your home that you either:

   1) Don't currently do at all, or
   2) Don't do regularly

This activity should be something that you would like to have done but are not really "thrilled" to do. (That is most likely why it is not being done!) Some examples might be making your bed every morning, going to sleep with the sink and kitchen area clean, vacuuming, or emptying the trash every night. There are many others... you decide on one. It is important that this activity is not vitally important to you in the overall fulfillment of your day. Write the activity on the line below:

My activity is:

Should you accept this challenge, the activity you chose will be practiced **every day for thirty consecutive days.** This is the challenge! Did you know that most people are unable to do anything new for much more than three days? I don't care if it is flossing their teeth or going to the gym, the average person cannot keep with a new activity for more than three days! What about you? I know you think you can, but have you ever acted on that thought?

The main objective of this challenge is to pick a simple activity that you will practice doing each day via repetition to see what forming a habit feels like. In order to become fulfilled in any area, you deserve to know what it feels like on an emotional level. For example: let's say you choose the task of making your bed each morning. It does not matter if you "want to" make your bed every day… that's not the point. The point is to see if you can actually, consciously do something new which is not routine for thirty consecutive days.

Liking the task is not a factor. You do not have to like exercising. You do not have to like networking. A "superstar" athlete does not have to like shooting four hundred free throws. In fact, there are many things that we don't like that will produce the results we do like. **The fulfilled person is willing to do what the average person is not.**

If you can do this new task for thirty consecutive days, I will guarantee you that by the last week it will be virtually effortless. When the thirty days are up, it will actually be hard *not* to do that task! This is a habit. The reason you should pick a task that is not vitally important to your overall fulfillment in life is that if you can repeat an action with a simple, unimportant task that has little meaning to the overall quality of your life, you can do it with anything.

Because an activity like making your bed is not as scary if you fail to do it, we essentially take fear and necessity of success out of the picture. Now you simply must rely on conscious thought and action to be successful at this. That's all it really takes to create a new habit

Tips to enhance your odds of success for this challenge

You must set yourself up for success. If you try and go through your thirty days without sharing what you are doing with anyone or not posting signs around the house saying, "Go make your bed," it will be more difficult to succeed. If you have no accountability, it will be too easy to miss a day and say at the end, "I missed a couple of days, but overall I did it." **With this challenge, you either do it or you don't... no "kind ofs."**

Your family can remind you each day and offer support in other ways. Just be sure you are clear what you want from them in terms of support so there is no conflict. Sharing with your family about what you are setting out to do is nice; however, you might require something more. Create incentives for your success or lack thereof. For instance, you can choose an incentive such as a massage or a weekend without the kids when you successfully complete your thirty days. If you do not complete the thirty days, think of something that you really *don't* want to do and put it on the line. This will act as a much-needed motivation when you feel like giving up.

Philosophy #3:

Fulfillment Is Not a Matter of Circumstance;
It Is Largely a Matter of Conscious Choice

Fulfillment is a conscious result; it is not a matter of luck, chance, or circumstances. Sure you can roll the dice and win, but then you are dealing with odds. You don't want to deal with odds when it comes to your life, because the odds are not in your favor… statistically, that's the way it is. You want to be in the driver's seat of your life and choose your own direction. Being in the driver's seat is not about control; it's about trust. Think about driving a car. Yes, you have control over the direction of the car, yet the trust comes from believing that the people driving in the opposite direction directly at you will not hit you head-on… *that is trust.*

In order to create unlimited wealth, you must know that you are only responsible for your fulfillment, and not the fulfillment of others. As an entrepreneur or career driven individual, you might be the leader of a team of employees, coworkers, or maybe a downline. If you are constantly feeling responsible for everyone else's fulfillment, you will tire very quickly by using unnecessary energy points. Be a great leader by leading yourself and role-modeling successful habits and disciplines. Show others how you are choosing to be fulfilled versus relying on outside sources to do it for you. Others can advise, tell, and coach, but in the end you and only you can consciously decide and seek answers from yourself.

These conscious decisions must come from a place in the heart of trust, not logic. Logic is where fear, doubt, insecurity, overwhelmed feelings, and your circumstances live. Circumstances are situations like your social status, race, ethnicity, financial, and health situation. Most people have been trained to allow these circumstances have the greatest influence over their decisions.

In some cases, this can be appropriate; however, when it comes to *Being Fulfilled*, using circumstances for its attainment will not work, because circumstances are derived from logic, and fulfillment is derived from emotion... two completely different sources. Succeeding from logic is like hunting in the woods with a fishing pole or deep-sea fishing with a shotgun.

> What would happen if we conducted an experiment where every time you wanted something in life and a circumstance of yours seemingly got in the way, we took care of it instantly? If your circumstance said you had no money... we gave you the money. No time... we created the time. No support... you received the support. I'm not just talking about material things, but rather the opportunities you are presented with daily where you choose to allow your circumstances to get in the way.
>
> In this experiment, by getting rid of the seemingly valid circumstance, we can now see a bit more clearly what is really holding you back. This is why when someone wants to hire me as a coach and says, "I don't have the money," I respond, "If you did have the money, would you hire me today?" If there is an instant yes, then I know they are allowing their circumstance to get in the way, and there is a deeper fear involved that is not letting them move forward.

> Everyone has "the money" or has access "to the money." They can earn it, borrow it, find it, or charge it. If your want is large enough, you never allow "the money," or another circumstance to get in your way.
>
> The next time you think a circumstance is stopping you from getting something, remember this experiment. Ask yourself, "If I did have 'X circumstance,' what would I do?" If you still are unable to decide and move forward into action, there is something else that is stopping you. At this point, acknowledge that it is not the circumstance but rather a fear or apprehension around something else. This is where coaching yourself (or working with one) will assist you in finding the true answers.

If you want become fulfilled, conscious choice is your ticket. You might think conscious choice is "thinking" and "logic"; however, conscious choice takes place in the heart, not the brain. Your heart is so much wiser than the brain. The brain is like the hard drive on a computer, a place where information and experiences are stored. Your heart is where decisions are created and conscious choice takes place. As humans, we use our emotions as keys to access the stored information in our brains. Emotions unlock our actions; logic applies the brakes.

Conscious choice is the same as what we term freedom of choice. Freedom of choice is essentially freedom of result. We are free to create whatever type of results we choose. Choosing is more powerful than wanting, because it is the first level of decision. Choosing boils down to your minute-by-minute decisions that take place inside your heart. When emotions or experiences seem too much to handle in the heart, people tend to bring their circumstances in to complicate things.

People complicate things so that they can validate an inner fear not to take action with an external circumstance. Example: A client, Dottie, wanted to release weight, but she kept saying she did not have the time to exercise and eat better. After some coaching we determined she *did have* the time to exercise but still was not taking action. Through more coaching, we uncovered her inner fear that if she lost all her weight she was afraid she would not want her husband anymore because he was overweight too. She feared she would be not attracted to him anymore and would wind up in a divorce, and that was painful to her. Bottom line, she stayed overweight and used the circumstance of lack of time as her excuse not to lose it.

Subconsciously, Dottie was not exercising because of a painful fear. In her heart, she wanted to become healthy and fit; however, there was a direct conflict between that value and the one she placed on her family and her husband. This is where her logic took over and began to complicate things. When Dottie recognized what was *really* holding her back, she consciously chose to release that fear, take action, and the weight started to fall off. So far she has released over forty pounds and is more in love than ever.

The next time you want to do something, or are presented with an opportunity and find your logic presenting circumstances as your reason *not* to proceed, take a moment to rid yourself of the circumstance and listen to your heart.

Philosophy #4:
Results Are Energy

Being fulfilled begins by understanding how we communicate with ourselves and with others. Communication is also known as connecting. This connection occurs when two people have something in common. Here is a basic flow on how *connecting* leads to *becoming fulfilled*.

Connecting = Relationships
Relationships = Influence
Influence = Decisions
Decisions = Results
Results = Unlimited Wealth
Unlimited Wealth = **Being Fulfilled**

This chart shows that being fulfilled begins by connecting with people. That connection will build a relationship over time. This time frame can be moments or years. Think of all the people you have great relationships with. Those relationships were born with a connection. The connection could be something in common, a similar experience you shared, or a feeling. Based on the nature of these relationships, you will have some level of trust with these people. The more trust you have, the better the relationships and the more influence you will have with them. Example: If my wife told me that I looked great in a pink suit, I would believe her more than the woman who was trying to sell it to me. My wife has much more influence over me than the saleswoman, because I trust her more.

BEING FULFILLED

The more influence you have with others, the greater the role you play in their decision creating process. Most people cannot decide for themselves. This is where you step in with all of your influence! With your influence, you can guide someone to a decision. Decisions are what create results. At the end of the day, unlimited wealth and being fulfilled is attained by creating desired results in business, relationships, and health. Because of this, it is paramount you understand how to connect.

How to Connect

You could be thinking one of two things: "Great! In order to create unlimited wealth and become fulfilled all I have to do is connect... I am a great connector!" or "Great... in order to create unlimited wealth and become fulfilled all I have to do is connect... I am a terrible connector." Please note that being a great connector does not guarantee your fulfillment by any means. There is so much more to the fulfillment equation than connecting; for instance, there are skills and systems that need to be learned. Connecting can start off as a skill, however, and when it's done effectively and effortlessly, it is an art. Skills you learn; arts you master. The goal here is to teach you the art of connecting so you can master it.

In order to be great at anything, at some point you must understand what it is and how it works. There are two ways you can understand processes: logically and intuitively. The process of connecting is not a logical process. Logic negates the very art of connecting. Example: If you are on a first date and you have a premade list of things you want to talk about, or if you are thinking too much about how to appropriately answer a question, trust me, there will be no connection and no second date. (Unless you are really cute!)

Connecting, like dating, is an intuitive process. It relies on trust and an openness to be in the moment and see the opportunities that present themselves. When you are in your head processing information, you are not present and you miss opportunities.

Seeking and Creating Opportunities

I was in California doing a seminar. I forgot something very important in my room and was rushing back to get it. At the time, I was working on being more in the moment, so I took a breath and opened up to possibility right before I walked on the elevator. I got on, hit the button for my floor, and instead of staring at the ground or at the floor indicator like most people do, I looked at each of the people on the elevator. One man was wearing a University of Massachusetts-Amherst shirt, which happens to be my alma mater. I said: "Did you graduate from UMass?" He looked up, gave me great eye contact, and said: "No, but my son goes there now." We began a brief conversation and then we arrived at his floor.

By this time I had learned that he was an entrepreneur who just sold his company and was exploring a new business venture. As he got off the elevator, I did too, and we continued the conversation, even though this was not my floor. He gave me all the signs of a great connection to have in my business, and I was not about to lose that connection because

> it was not my floor. The result was that we exchanged business cards, and two weeks later he purchased my eight-CD audio course, *Healthy Mind Healthy Body*. We still keep in touch, and I know that this connection will be valuable in the future. If I did not breathe before I got in that elevator, I would have been so in my head that I would not even have noticed this man.

In order to connect, you must relax. Relaxing sends out an attractive energy that people around you pick up on. Connection is created from the energy that comes within. Energy is the essence of how we communicate and form our relationships. Let me break down connecting through effective communication so you can see how it works:

Effective Communication Consists of:

7% Words
38% Tone
55% Energy

Energy Defined

It is clear to see that the spoken word means very little. We can all remember conversations with people where they went on and on while we checked out of the conversation. Our tone, which is how we say what we say, weighs a little more in effective communication. While these first two components have some importance, it is clear that the main ingredient in effective communication is energy. So what is energy?

Energy is not something tangible; it just is. If we were to simply break it down to a quantum level, deep within the cells of our body, energy is all those tiny molecules vibrating at a certain frequency. These molecules are so small that they are not even visible with a powerful microscope. That is tiny! Take a look at the book you are reading, the chair you are sitting on, and your left leg. Everything around us, including ourselves, is made up of the same elements: hydrogen, oxygen, nitrogen, and carbon… EVERYTHING!

Everything looks different because the molecules are in different forms; we call these bodies. In these unique bodies, each of these molecules vibrates at a different frequency. These different frequencies are being transmitted to the universe at all times in the form of energy. This energy can neither be created nor destroyed; it is simply exchanged.

Example: An ice cube is consistent with its vibration unless you do something to it, like heat it up. At this point it melts, boils, and evaporates. Eventually it will come back down as rain. By applying the heat, all you did was change the vibration of the molecules and they changed form. Ice and water are the same; the only difference is how the molecules are vibrating.

As humans, our molecules are constantly changing their vibration as we have different thoughts, feelings, and experiences. So at any given moment in our day, we can be sending off a completely different energy. This energy is transmitted and received by other people, because as humans, we are transmitters and receivers. As a transmitter, we send off energy into the universe based on our thoughts, feelings, and experiences. As receivers, we feel the energy that other people are transmitting.

Trusting the Energy

We receive energy from others using our receiving tools. These tools are our intuition, our gut feelings, and what people have labeled a "sixth sense." In order to become great at listening to these receiving tools, we must trust them. How well do you trust your instincts? How well do you trust those impulse feelings you receive in a situation? Have you ever said phrases like:

> *"I don't know what it is, but I don't like…"*
> *"Something smells fishy around here."*
> *"Something's different in the air."*
> *"I can't put my finger on it, but…"*
> *"There's something different about you."*
> *"I'm getting a bad vibe from this person/thing."*
> *"I am sensing there is something wrong."*

What you are referring to is the energy you are receiving around a person or an event. The great part about energy is that *energy cannot lie.* Look once again at the ingredients of effective communication:

7% Words
38% Tone
55% Energy

Our words and tone can lie, but our energy cannot. Here's an example: Have you ever had a friend come to visit and as soon as she walked in the door, you could feel that something was wrong? Even though she was "pretending" to be herself, you sensed something was wrong. You ask, "What's wrong?" She says, "Nothing." You ask again, "Come on, what's wrong?" and she still says, "Nothing!" Heck, your dog knew something was wrong! No matter what she says or how she says it, it does not mask the fact that she is not herself. If she is open enough, she might eventually admit that something is happening. This is when you can say: "See, I knew it!" Bottom line… energy cannot lie.

Becoming Attractive

Jim Rohn says that in order to attract success, you must become an attractive person. In order to attract the right type of people in your life, you must become attractive. Not attractive like Adonis, but attractive from an energy standpoint. Everyone is attracting something into their life; however, is it what they want? Remember, we *receive* energy from others using our receiving tools. As for the energy we *transmit* at any given time, it is important to remember that this is influenced by our thoughts, feelings, and experiences. Knowing how all this energy is coming and going, how and what does our energy attract?

This is commonly referred to as The Law of Attraction, which boils down to this: like energy attracts like energy. This is an easy way to show how your results work. The law of attraction is vibrational energy transmitted by how you feel.

Let's use you and I as an example. Let's say you are feeling sad, so the molecules in your body are vibrating at a certain frequency. For the sake of learning, let's call this sad frequency "twenty." When you are feeling sad, your body transmits a "twenty" signal to the universe. On the other hand, I am feeling amazing. When I feel amazing, the molecules in my body are vibrating at a certain frequency; let's call this amazing frequency "two hundred."

Here is the scene: You and I are at a party. We both walk in the door at the same time. I am sending off my amazing "two hundred" energy and you are pumping out your sad "twenty." The question is: Who and what are we each going to attract?

I would guarantee that by the end of the night, I will be having an amazing time with all the people in the room that connected with my "two hundred" energy. You will be having a sad time with the people that connected with your "twenty" energy. We cannot deny that like attracts like. You will be connecting with a different type of person that evening, because that is the energy you are sending out.

You and I will not connect, because we will have nothing to talk about; we cannot relate to each other. You will want to complain about your day, whereas I would be on a high from my day. Not only does your sad energy attract sad people, but it also allows you to notice more sad events.

There is a line from a Jimmy Durante song that says, "Put on a happy face." In the case of the law of attraction, think about it like putting on a pair of 3-D glasses. Whatever mood you are in determines what type of lenses you look through. When you are sad, you put on your 3-D sad glasses. When you have on your 3-D sad glasses, what pops out? All the sad things! You begin to hit all the red lights while you are late for an appointment. The people next to you on the beach light up their cigarettes and you hate smoke. You are eating lunch and the ketchup from your burger drips on your new white shirt.

When you have on your 3-D sad glasses, you become even sadder and say, "Just what I expected!" or "This always happens to me." You'll often hear people say "when one thing goes wrong, everything goes wrong." This is not the case. What went wrong is that you put on your 3-D sad glasses and never took them off. Now everything you see is sad, because that is all the 3-D sad glasses will point out for you.

You may be asking, "So, by being sad, did I attract these events?" You did not attract those events; you simply noticed and focused on them more because of the energy state you were in. These events will have happened whether you were there or not. You can be in an amazing mood and still hit every red light, or be next to the smokers on the beach and drop the ketchup on your shirt. The difference is that when you are feeling amazing, you're wearing your 3-D amazing glasses.

The same events happen; however, you will see them differently. You see the red lights as an opportunity to roll down the windows, open the sunroof, and enjoy the ride to the appointment. With your 3-D amazing glasses on, when people light up the cigarettes on the beach, you simply get up and go for a walk or move your spot. When the ketchup drips on your shirt, you laugh and make a joke of it. You say things like, "Everything is coming up roses" and "I'm on a roll." You feel like everything is lining up and falling into place.

BEING FULFILLED

The people you have attracted into your world are there because at some point you connected with their energy and them with yours. Specific events and happenings in your world are present no matter if you feel happy or sad. What you *choose* to see depends on what feeling 3-D glasses you are wearing at any given moment. Remember when I got on the elevator where I met the man with the University of Massachusetts-Amherst shirt on? He was going to be on that elevator no matter how I was feeling. *I did not attract him to the elevator; we were attracted to each other on the elevator.* There is a big difference.

I was able to see and connect with him because before I got on that elevator I consciously chose to change the pair of 3-D glasses I was wearing—from frantic and rushing to relaxed and open. If I boarded the elevator with my 3-D frantic glasses on, I might have connected with the other person who was nervously tapping his foot and letting out a disgusted sigh every time there was a delay. Because I chose to put on my 3-D relaxed glasses, I actually resisted that person tapping his foot and said in my mind, "What's his problem?"

Attraction Is a Choice

All of this ties in intimately with Philosophy #3: *Fulfillment is not a matter of circumstance; it is largely a matter of conscious choice.* Attraction is a choice. It is about you choosing how you want to feel and what type of results you want. Who do you want to be around? Just because you entered the party sad, with a "twenty" energy level, does not mean you cannot leave with an amazing "two hundred" feeling. Attraction is not about hoping, wishing, dreaming, or praying that something will change. Attraction simply increases your odds of achieving the results you seek in a relaxed, steady state.

Be sure you understand that just thinking positively will not get you the results you desire. This goes back to the statement made earlier about the man on the elevator. *I did not attract him to the elevator; we were attracted to each other on the elevator.* My being in an open mood is what attracted us to each other. After that attraction took place, it was up to me to close the deal. Never discount the bold, consistent action required to achieve results. *Attraction is the first step.* Once the attraction takes place, then you must utilize the skills, knowledge, and other tools you have developed to obtain the result.

Once I got off the elevator with that man, I used the listening, asking, and closing skills that I have worked hard on to seal the deal. My result was a $150 sale and a great connection for possible future results. Attraction did not do that for me; it was only the first step. **I was responsible** after that.

Coach's Challenge

The first step to achieving bigger results is to create an awareness of where you are and what you are doing. This challenge is based on the concept of the 3-D glasses shared in this philosophy.

The Challenge

Find—or purchase—three pairs of 3-D glasses. If they are not 3-D, who cares, just make sure they are big, funny looking, and colorful. It doesn't matter where you get them or how cheap they are. The main point is that they are very odd and funny looking… not ones you would feel comfortable wearing in public.

Strategically put these glasses in places you invest lots of time in. Maybe put a pair on your office desk, a pair next to your nightstand, and a pair on the counter in your kitchen. The next time you are in an undesirable mood or your day is not going the way you would like it to… go find the glasses. Put the glasses on, look in the mirror, and ask yourself: "What mood am I looking through these lenses with?" Don't hold back from laughing at yourself, but really try and identify what mood you are in and why. Ask yourself, "If I choose to stay this mood for the rest of the day, how will this impact my results?"

Just by putting on the glasses, you will increase the odds of changing your mood and perspective. When you do this enough, not only will your mood change, but your results will too! Having these glasses in highly visible places will allow them to become constant, empowering triggers that will remind you of the mood you are in and the messages you learned about in this philosophy.

The Objective

The objective is to allow yourself to become more consciously aware of *why* you are experiencing *what* you are experiencing. Remember, your results have to do with how you feel and the glasses you are looking through. Essentially, by putting on the glasses you are pressing PAUSE to the mood you are in. Putting your mood on pause creates an opportunity for you to realize how that mood could affect the rest of your day, week, or even month if you don't consciously choose to change it.

Please note that you do not *have to* change your mood at this point. You may determine that being mad is appropriate for the time being. The difference is that now you are *choosing* to be mad, so you have command over your emotions. Now your mood is on purpose versus out of control. You don't want to bury an emotion; you want to release it. You must determine if you can release it now, or if it requires more time.

It is very important to have glasses that are funny and wild. This will break the normal patterns in your mood and allow you to easily shift your association in the moment. When you are beginning the process of creating new behaviors, tangible reminders and rituals like this are absolutely necessary for success. These rituals break the associations and bad feelings you become addicted to that keep you doing the same things over and over again.

It's up to you who you wish to include in this process. The more people you include in this process, when appropriate, the better your odds are for success. If these people are supportive, once they understand what you are doing, you will benefit greatly by having them involved. Your relationships will also grow closer because of this teamwork and support network.

Please recognize that some people will be supportive and others will not. You must determine who and when it's appropriate to bring someone into this process. Never use people that are not supportive as an excuse not to do this. In the end, even if you have a large support network, fulfillment is your choice.

Success Story

One of my coaching clients who did this challenge used her husband very effectively. She gave him *permission* to use these glasses when he felt she was "in a mood." Whenever he sensed she was in a mood, he would go put the glasses on her... and he put on a pair too! He would pull her over to a mirror while saying, "Remember, you asked me for my assistance and gave me permission to do this!" They began laughing together, she changed her mood, their relationship blossomed, and she created massive results by releasing lots of weight and seeing her business profits soar!

By putting the glasses on and changing her mood, she broke old patterns that would put her into a depression for months. Imagine if you were upset and all of a sudden someone you gave permission to turned around with these crazy glasses on? How might that change your results?

Philosophy #5:
When You Judge Yourself Less and Trust More You Will have Everything You Want

"Never judge a book by its cover," so they say. It's too bad that in the real world this does not work. People *do* judge a book by its cover, and they will judge you, too. You cannot help if others judge you, but you can release your judgment upon yourself. When you judge yourself less, you will have more of what you want…. In fact, **when you judge yourself less and trust more, you will find out that everything you ever wanted… you already have!**

When you become judgment free, you are objective. This objectivity detaches you from labels like good, bad, positive, or negative. Everything in life is what it is—in other words, a result is a result. Being objective with yourself allows you to detach from your situation and essentially become an observer. This could be described as an out-of-body experience. When you are detached, you essentially become your own guide and consciousness. You are able to see things the way they are and have less reactive emotion attached to them. The less reactive you become, the more aware and open you are to noticing the opportunities that come your way.

When you come from an authentic place versus judging a situation, you are unattached to a specific outcome and are more likely to take fearless action. Fear does not exist, because fear is derived from judgment. It will feel like an internal wisdom propels your actions, and those actions become effortless. You act from the heart and from your well-established values. Now you feel like you have a reason for being, a clear life purpose, and you know what you are here for. This is called fulfillment, and it's where unlimited wealth begins.

The end result is that you become very present to who you are. You do not have to think about who you are, because your presence is always there. In this objective place, you come from a deeper knowing of who you are. Your self-esteem soars, and this is the point where you get more mileage from your ten energy points. When you embrace a judgment free life, you live with fewer hang-ups and concerns.

There are many qualities that people desire to possess—patience, love, and feeling carefree. These qualities are only found in a world without judgment. To love unconditionally means to love without judgment. To be carefree, to speak and act from what you truly feel does not have judgment attached to it. To be patient and allow life to flow and take its natural course requires focused objectivity.

In the legal system, everyone is innocent until proven guilty. However, some people treat themselves like they are guilty until proven innocent. They say: "I am not lovable"; "I am not good enough"; "I am bad at this"; and "Why am I so stupid?" This is how people judge themselves.

Trust will free you of judgment. **Trust is your biggest lever of resources... time and energy.** When you lack trust, you must do so much more work to get the same job done. For instance, when was the last time you asked someone to do something for you? Were you checking up on them constantly while they were doing it? Did you double-check the result they produced "just to make sure" it was done correctly? This demonstrates a lack of trust of others and yourself.

When you trust yourself in a higher, judgment free zone, you do not censor what you want to say and how you wish to act. Have you ever thought, "They are not going to like the sound of that?" When we censor our actions and words, we are trying to protect ourselves and others from something we are judging to be painful. Most people fear that someone will reject what they say or do. Because of the judgment, they become diplomatic... where does that get them?

Diplomacy is trying to say the truth without having to say the truth. It is a form of peacekeeping and a tiptoe feeling. It is okay and sometimes appropriate to be diplomatic with others, but how diplomatic are you with yourself? How do you dance around what you deserve to hear? Until you put the laser beam upon yourself, the truth will never be seen. In one of his movies, Jack Nicholson said, "You can't handle the truth." When you cease believing that, the truth *will* set you free.

Trusting allows you to know at a deeper level. Knowing enables you to act more from your heart and stay away from logic, which, as I've said, lies in your head. This philosophy ties in directly with the third one: Fulfillment is not a matter a circumstance; it is largely a matter of conscious choice. Acting from a place of trust enables you to choose more quickly and see results sooner. Trust can be developed and cultivated. It stems from your internal messages and is created from within. Once you identify the judgmental messages that inhibit trust, you can create new messages and begin the three-step process of change discussed earlier.

Exercise

Take a piece of paper and draw a six-inch horizontal line from left to right. On the left side of the line draw a minus sign (-) and on the right side of the line draw a plus sign (+). Under the minus sign, write down five negative emotions that you experience on a fairly regular basis. Under the plus sign, write down five positive emotions you experience on a regular basis. Do this before you read any further.

Below is an example:

(-) -------------------------------- (+)	
Guilt	Joy
Overwhelmed	Laughter
Frustration	Excitement
Anger	Relief
Envy	Lov

Which side took you longer to come up with five emotions? If you are like most people, you rattled off the negative ones quickly and had to think a bit more about five positive ones. This is just an illustration of how we are conditioned to focus on negative aspects of life.

Now look at both sides of the line. Pick any of your negative emotions and any of the positive ones and think of the physical effects each has on your body. If you look at it objectively, each and every emotion, positive or negative, has virtually the same physical effects on your body. Each causes your heart rate to increase, releases adrenaline, slows digestion, opens your capillaries, and makes you more alert. Your body does not see these emotions as good or bad, it responds the same either way.

We are the ones who judge an emotion as good or bad. Why does anger have to be bad? Have you ever felt great being angry? Has guilt ever led you in a more appropriate direction? Has love ever hurt and joy caused pain? The point of this exercise is to show that the only difference between a negative emotion like guilt and a positive one like joy is how we judge them.

The objective here is to strip away any judgment around your emotions and re-label them as simply emotions. An emotion is nothing more than a signal from your body telling you something is happening. If you stub your toe on a door frame, the pain is helpful so you don't do it again. That pain you feel is not bad, but rather a signal from your toe saying, "Hey… don't do that again." If that pain were not there, one day you might look down and see a few toes missing!

The next time you feel any emotion, ask yourself: "What signal is my body trying to send me? What is the cause of this emotion? How do I usually act when I experience this emotion? What actions are appropriate for me to express now? What actions can I take to release or enhance this feeling? How can I prevent this from happening again so I don't arrive at this place again?" These questions assume the emotion is not good or bad but simply a signal. It allows you to respond versus react. Doing this with "positive" emotions is just as important. Most people when they feel great have no idea how they arrived there or how to get back. These questions allow you to have a higher level of consciousness about what you are feeling and why.

Philosophy #6:
Perfection Does Not Exist

You know the old saying, "Practice makes perfect?" Let me tell you, **practice does not make perfect... practice makes you better**. All you perfectionists out there are resisting right now; however, you know this is true. As a coach I have asked literally hundreds of people in seminars and my clients, "Are you a perfectionist?" Most say yes. Then I ask, "Do you believe perfection is possible?" Almost everyone will say no. What they are really saying is *"No, I do not believe perfection is possible, yet I constantly struggle for something I don't believe I can get, so I keep failing and proving my belief that perfection is not possible correct."*

When you strive for something that you truly do not believe is possible, like perfection, a habit is formed... a failing habit. If you keep on the cycle of struggling and failing, struggling and failing, you are essentially practicing that cycle. You become very familiar with that cycle, and you get addicted to those feelings because that is all you know. Because humans instinctually gravitate towards situations that are familiar, after a while all you know how to do is struggle and fail... and you actually begin to like it!

In order to break this cycle, begin to recognize that perfection is at best 80 percent. This will allow you to release the 100% syndrome and strive for your best. Let's call this "80 percent perfect." With 80 percent perfect, you do your best and move on. The way you achieve unlimited wealth is by doing your best and moving on. You don't achieve a result by doing the same thing over and over trying to make it better and better. When you strive for this kind of perfection, 100% perfection, you never finish and are never really satisfied with your work. 100% perfection is a cycle that will teach you how to fail.

Take this book for example. I can write and rewrite. I can proofread and revise. I could do this literally for years. At the end of the day, I would be frustrated, unfulfilled, and not have a published book... hence, no result.

The 80 percent perfect philosophy allows you to perform your actions to the best of your ability. Just like writing books—write it, proof it, print it, sell it... end of story! Will it be perfect? Eighty percent perfect! There may be some sentences that make no sense, or maybe even a speelling error! Some of you analytical people are freaking out right now. *"Oh my God, he has a misspelled word!"* The point is, 80 percent perfect allows you to attain a result that you can be proud of and reap the rewards versus struggling with no results. If someone has a problem with a misspelled word or a grammatically incorrect sentence, whose perfection issue is it... theirs or mine?

This 80 percent perfect philosophy releases pressure so you can produce a result and not worry about everything being 100% perfect. If you can honestly say that you did the best you could, took all the necessary steps that were in your ability to do, can you be happy with the result? This philosophy is designed to get you up and moving. Most people wait until they are ready.... When does that happen? NEVER. Eighty percent perfect acknowledges that you are already ready!

While 80 percent perfection is important, realize that there are places where 100% perfection is required. A civil engineer who designs a bridge that millions pass over each day better be 100% perfect. Here exact precision is an absolute must. However, when it comes to being an entrepreneur or career driven individual who is growing a business, seeking better health, and forming solid relationships, your results rely on massive action, not getting ready to get ready and blaming it on perfection.

If you remember the last philosophy about releasing judgment, perfection is only a judgment of being good enough for your own standards, or worse yet, someone else's. Not only is perfection a judgment, but it is a moving target as well. It is not letting anybody see *what you judge* to be a weakness. Doing something so well, to a level of perfection, is part of a camouflage so people cannot see a perceived weakness. This is something you don't want them to see, so you work so hard at an image of you that is not truthful.

You don't have to be everything to everybody; you just have to be something to yourself. If you are not sure what that something is, then you are always working on creating the camouflage called perfection.

The end result is being frozen in procrastination. Years go by while you are trying to figure out what "good enough" is, but you never find it. **"Good enough" is who you already are, not who you are trying to become**. This last statement must be true, or else no one could ever be good enough. When you accept that you are "good enough" as you are now, it will release all the pressure—because striving for perfection is exhausting. People in an exhausting relationship get out of it. You are in a relationship with yourself that you must be in. If that relationship is exhausting, you will end up hating yourself.

Philosophy #7:
Fear of Success Is Greater than Fear of Failure

Most people who never get started will blame their procrastination on fear. When asked, what are you afraid of, most reply, "Fear of failure." While fear of failure can be real in a given situation, the foundation of this philosophy rests upon a simple fact that the fear of success, in most cases, is the main cause of procrastination.

Here's why. Fear is caused by unknown, unfamiliar, uncertain, and uncharted territory. Fear essentially is caused mostly by something you have not experienced much, if ever, in your life. When it comes to failure, though, this is a known. Everyone has failed before. Whether it was a test, a goal, or a relationship, we have all experienced the defeat and disappointment that failure brings.

So the real question is, "If you have failed so many times in the past, what is so unfamiliar and uncertain about the feeling of failure?" It sounds like you have been quite familiar with it from your past. How can someone be so afraid of something they know so well? Because of this familiarity with failure, the real point here is that fear of failure does not exist.

Success, on the other hand, is something rarer. We have all have had the sweet taste of victory and felt the empowering emotions of the win. What happens after the win? As humans, it is our nature to want more and to grow. It is a physiological fact that we are either growing or dying. The processes in your body that builds you up are called anabolic, and the ones that break you down are called catabolic. Because of this growing or dying nature, the quest to have, do, be, and see is intrinsic. This is why everyone is looking for a better business, better relationship, and better health.

BEING FULFILLED

Taking the necessary steps in the pursuit of the next level of success is absolutely an unknown, no matter what level of success you are seeking. You can read a book on success, talk to a mentor who has "been there and done that," or attend a seminar on how to do what you are seeking, but at the end of the day, your journey to this new level is unique, uncharted, unfamiliar, and because of this… scary! This is called fear of success.

You look at successful people and think, "I could never do what they do." "If that is what it takes to succeed, I don't want to." "What will I have to change and sacrifice to get to that level?" "What type of pace will I have to maintain to stay at that new level once there?"

The fact is, failure is easy and success is not. It is easy to settle and remain in the status quo. It is hard to put yourself on the line and expect more from yourself and others. It is easy to be cloaked in failure, because everywhere you look, someone is complaining about *their* failures. It is hard to be consistent, patient, and focused when you are seemingly sailing into unknown areas and not seeing any immediate results.

So why is everyone blaming their procrastination on fear of failure when it is clearly the easy path and very familiar to them? I wouldn't spend too much time on this; however, that is exactly what many people do: they spend too much time studying their failures.

Which are you better at, success or failure? Your answer boils down to the amount of time you spend studying each of them. Most people are very proficient at failure, even though they want success so badly. They spend so much time going over what went wrong and why it happened by breaking it down, analyzing it, and asking questions like, "Why am I so bad?" "What is wrong with me?" "Why does this always happen to me?"

Because of this, failing becomes so familiar that fear is nothing more than a jargon word they use to make them feel better as to why they are not taking action. Are you getting so good at researching your failures and disappointments that you have earned your master's degree in failing? Remember, what you focus on grows.

When was the last time you succeeded and sat down to figure out what went right and why it happened? When have you asked questions like, "What allowed me to perform so well?" "What strengths did I utilize most effectively for this win?" Most people will create a victory, celebrate it, and very quickly move on to the next "to do" item on their list. When you spend most of your time understanding your victories, the fear of success begins to subside because you understand success more. It will not take long before you have your bachelor's degree in success and will be well on your way to your master's!

Let's Get Honest—Fear Is Not the Cause

Come on, let's cut through the lies you tell yourself and own up to the truth. While the fear of failure or success can have an influence on your decisions, fear is a jargon word that people use as a crutch. Whether you have a fear of failure or a fear of success, fear is the effect, not the cause. You might think that risk is the cause of fear, but all risk implies is that you do not believe. **There is no risk when you believe.** If something is too risky or scary, it is only because you lack belief. In other words, you do not trust beyond a shadow of a doubt. Take a look at this:

1% Doubt = 0% Trust
0% Doubt = 100% Trust

BEING FULFILLED

Have you ever heard the saying, "Beyond the shadow of a doubt?" Have you ever wondered *what* is beyond the shadow of a doubt? It's a word we have discussed called trust. If you doubt, even a shadow, even .0001%, your odds of failure are increased. And from this shadow of doubt stems procrastination and self-sabotage. As you can see, when you trust 100%, there is no doubt, fear, or risk… just pure reward and fulfillment.

Why People Procrastinate and Sabotage their Progress

Why people procrastinate and sabotage their progress is not as mysterious as it may seem. Take an honest look at the cause of procrastination, and see if you can be open enough to objectively listen to what you read and begin to apply it to yourself. If you read and connect with the information, but do not own up to the fact that this is what is going on, you will remain stuck.

Let's set the scenario. You are working really hard, trying so hard to make ends meet by working hour after hour. Things begin to get a little scary and a bit too hard. At this point, you really want to give up, but that is not acceptable. What would people say and think? You conjure up all these reasons to quit; no time, no money, no resources, and you are scared… the list in your head goes on and on. But *really*, you cannot believe these excuses; these are not valid reasons to stop.

This is where you begin to subconsciously, or worse yet, consciously sabotage yourself by making things harder than they really are. For instance, you work out and eat well all week and then blow it on the weekend. You go to networking meeting after meeting and finally receive some leads, but you do not call them back or follow through. Essentially you are taking the long route when you know there is a better way; you are throwing tacks on the road to blow your own tires.

This cycle of trying so hard and failing… trying so hard and failing… begins to wear you out. You become physically and emotionally exhausted. This is what the saying "burning the candle at both ends" means. One end is physical and the other emotional. After a time period of enough internal resistance and pain… tying so hard and exhaustion… it happens. You are at the end of your rope and have a breakdown. Bottom line, you are done.

At this point, you *literally* cannot do any more, because you are emotionally and physically trash. This is where sabotage transitions from excuse to reason. Now you *can* stop and quit because there is a real, believable reason to quit: you are so exhausted. This works because *there is no guilt in honest exhaustion*. Think about the day you call in sick from work because you have a stomach virus. You don't lie in bed guilty when you are *really* sick.

People sabotage their success so they have a real reason to quit. This exhaustion creates a valid reason to stay in their comfort zone and not have to put themselves out there to try new things, not have to change. When they are asked why they didn't stay in the game, they can proudly say: "I was sick; I just could not handle the stress; it was physically and emotionally too much for me." People on the other end will say: "Tell me about it!"

You begin to create reasons, like stress and exhaustion, which validate what you expected to happen in the first place… the fact that you would not succeed. Essentially, you are proving yourself right! For example: Deep down you knew, based on past experience, that you would not succeed at what you are setting out to do. Because you hate to be wrong, in order to save your precious ego, you prove the expectation that you would not succeed to be right by sabotaging yourself. In the end you *are* right! You *are* a failure; you *are* not good enough and do *not* deserve success, just as you predicted and expected. In a very awkward yet comforting way, you are happy in your misery. It might sound silly when you read it or say it out loud, but it is the truth. Hence the saying: "Misery loves company."

My Friend of Misery

There is a song by Metallica called *My Friend of Misery*. Read the lyrics to see what you connect with.

You just stood there screaming, fearing no one was listening to you... they say the empty can rattles the most, the sound of your own voice must sooth you... hearing what you only want to hear, and knowing only what you heard, YOU... you're smothered in tragedy, yet you're off to save the world.

Misery... you insist that the weight of the world should be on your shoulders, Misery... there's much more than life than what you see... my friend of misery.

You still stood there screaming, no one caring about these words you tell, my friend before your

> *voice is gone... one man's fun is another's hell... these times they seem to try men's souls, but something's wrong with all you see... YOU, you'll take it on all yourself... Remember, Misery loves company!*
>
> *Misery... you insist that the weight of the world should be on your shoulders, Misery... there's much more than life than what you see... my friend of misery.*
>
> Poetry is powerful! When you really begin to understand what these lyrics are saying, you will begin to unravel why you do what you do.

Everyone has sabotaged their progress at one time or another. The objective here is to heighten your awareness of when you are in these situations so you don't become an expert at failing. Once you are more aware, you want to ask yourself questions to discover the why. Not the external why—but the one inside you really don't want to admit. This way you can stop blaming fear and get to the real cause.

Philosophy #8:

Balance as you Know It Does Not Exist and Is Not Necessary

If there has ever been a word that has been more misunderstood, "balance" would rank up there with the best of them. In today's world, it seems that everyone is seeking balance in all areas of their life, yet I have never met anyone who has actually achieved it... or at least had it for very long. This elusive goal of balance can be very alluring yet frustrating to attain. What is balance anyway? When I have asked many clients of mine that question, I have never received a clear answer. What is your definition of balance?

Balance is:_____

_____

_____

Most people define balance as all parts being equal, steadiness in life, poise, and stability. Based on that answer, it seems obvious why so many are seeking this state of being. It seems clear from these definitions that balance is not something external, but rather it's an internal state and overall feeling of stability. How did your definition match up to the one described here? If most people's definition confirms the need and quest for balance, why is it so difficult to achieve?

After defining balance in words, I asked many clients and seminar participants to draw visually what balance looked like for them. In the space below, draw your visual representation of what balance looks like to you. Feel free to draw more than one representation.

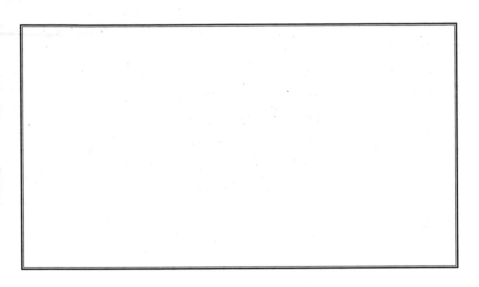

Now that you have your visual, here is what others drew:

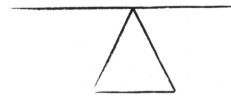

Other visuals included someone balancing on a tightrope, a set of balancing scales like the ones seen in the judicial system, and a seesaw leveled off. Look back to your written definition of balance and the one presented here of being in a state of stability, poise, and steadiness in life. How congruent is your written definition with your visual? Look at some of the visuals again

BEING FULFILLED

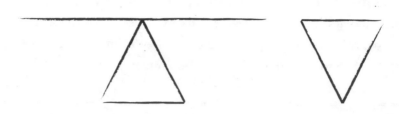

How stable and steady are these images? Not to stable at all. The reason many people do not achieve balance is because there is a huge contradiction between what they think it is supposed to be, how they envision it to look, and how they are trying to achieve it. This leads to the philosophy that balance as you know it does not exist. Balance *as you know* it is like trying to juggle many balls at once. **Let's redefine balance by using the word "stable," which would be like holding one ball.**

As I covered in the first section of the book, we only have ten energy points each day to give. The only way to be truly fulfilled and achieve unlimited wealth is by focusing on ONE AREA (one ball) for a long period of time. In order to do that, you must put down all the other "balls" you were previously juggling and focus on just one. Because you are no longer holding multiple "balls," you no longer require the need for balance. The need for balance assumes that you have two or more "balls." When you have one "ball"... one focus... it is always in balance. One focus is always stable, where many are less stable.

Knowing you no longer require balance, what does that feel like? How will this feeling allow you to be more productive and get more from your ten energy points? Most of my clients described achieving balance as feeling like they were walking on a tightrope. Once they focused on one area and put all their "balls" down, they described the feeling as if they jumped off the tightrope and had both feet touching the ground. You cannot take a step forward and take action until you are grounded.

Philosophy #9:
Become Focused, Not Busy

Today, all you hear is people telling you how busy they are. They say things like, "I am so crazy busy I cannot get anything done." It seems funny that someone is so busy but is not accomplishing anything. Based on that statement, it is clear that being busy does not produce desired results.

Busy is defined as being fully occupied in a particular activity. If you look in the thesaurus for the word busy, you will find words like demanding, hard, tiring, hectic, and empty. According to these words, being busy does not produce a result; it just keeps you shuffling papers around and tires you out.

There is a big difference between being busy and being focused. Have you ever heard someone say, "I am so focused that I cannot get anything done?" Focus is defined as having a concentrated effort and attention on a specific area. Look in the thesaurus under focus and you will find words like center, heart, center of attention, hub, and focal point. When you are focused, you will produce a desired result with a lot less effort, time, and energy. Based on only having ten energy points each day to give, adopting the ability to focus is a vital component to unlimited wealth and being fulfilled.

It's up to you to know when you are busy versus focused. Typically, when you are trying to do, be, and see everything in life, you are not focused, and you wind up tired and unfulfilled. If you are juggling too many balls (in this case, more than one) you will most likely find yourself busy all the time to keep them in the air. Using Philosophy #8 and understanding that balance is not necessary will assist you in becoming more focused.

You can better understand the difference between the two by taking a closer look at the activities in your day. What specifically are you accomplishing each day? How well do those specific accomplishments line up with what is required of you to be fulfilled in that area of focus? How often are you distracted, and what is distracting you?

Being distracted easily and often is a great signal that you are busy, but not focused. A lack of focus distracts you because you have no idea what you are doing next. Honestly, how have your results been this calendar year? How would your results change with a consistent focus? What would it take to weed out all the fluff in your life and find a focus so you can experience true fulfillment?

Philosophy #10:
Act Before You Think

Achieving extraordinary results is accomplished by challenging all the rules of life and taking action from a trusting place. What if you grew up hearing the opposite of everything?

- *Rock the boat*
- *It is easier done than said*
- *Act before you think*

- *Put yourself before others*
- *Rome was built in a day*
- *Receiving is better than giving*

How would your current results change? Playing by the rules is important when it comes to the law, sporting events, and board games; however, this is not the situation when it comes to being fulfilled. It's not that all the rules work against you, but rather to challenge all the rules to discover if they assist or resist your results. One of the biggest rules that society has adopted is thinking before you act. In many situations, thinking is very appropriate and necessary. When it comes to true fulfillment however, thinking will steer you away and cloud your vision from your authentic path.

It may not make sense logically to back out of a deal, relationship, or opportunity; however, if you want to honor your gut feelings and sleep at night, you'd better stop thinking and act from a place of inner trust. This inner trust acknowledges that you know yourself better than anyone else can. Only you know if you really want to do something or not. I'm not talking about things like running on the treadmill, hard conversations, or cold calling... those are things we don't like to do that we know are necessary for fulfillment. I'm talking about emotional situations and social contracts that pull you away from your focus and unnecessarily drain your energy points.

Remember, fear, doubt, insecurity, and overwhelmed feelings reside in your head where thought and logic come from. Because of this, **when you act without thinking, anything is possible; when you think before you act, what is possible is limited by your fears, doubts, and insecurities.**

BEING FULFILLED

People have been duped into believing that they require safety and security in life. They have been duped into thinking that having a steady job and carefully considering everything will allow them fulfillment. Just how safe, secure, and fulfilling is having a steady paycheck and health insurance? Most people in that position live paycheck to paycheck and often use phrases like: "I don't have the money"; "I don't have the time"; "Let me think about it"; and "I am trying to make ends meet."

Acting without thinking gives you the ability and potential to create more safety, security, and fulfillment than you could ever dream of, because your dreams can be as big as you wish. Walt Disney, Michael Dell, and J.K. Rowling are great examples of that. Allowing your thoughts to control your results is like a prison... you might as well be dead. When you take the leap of faith and trust your inner compass, the result will be unlimited wealth and being fulfilled.

Prison Break

Living in your head, being guided by logic, is like being in prison. If you have any desire to escape from that prison, you'd better do it quickly when the guards aren't looking and when everyone is sleeping. Your logic is the jail of your dreams. Your dream is looking to escape and become liberated from pain and fear. You've got to make a break for it, when logic least expects it. Once you make your attempt for the prison break and the alarms are blaring, the guards are running and the spotlights are shining, there's no going back. You've made your commitment, and

---

now, you either go for it all or go back to jail with another strike against you and a longer sentence. Are you in or out? It's a higher sense of decision.

When you act from passion and heart, you have a natural adrenaline rush. Once you have the adrenaline, you must not stop, think, or slow down, because the adrenaline will wear off. When you feel a spark inside of you, this is the time to act. A spark is something inside of you that cannot be matched. Sparks are created from dreams that connect and align every cell in our body.

This situation cannot be created by logic. This is called inspiration, which produces enthusiasm. Enthusiasm literally means "the God within." The only thing that can extinguish this flame that you have created is your logic. Logic is the terminator of all dreams. It's the fire extinguisher of hope. It's the blanket that smothers the fire. It's the shower that rained on the parade. Logic is the static coming through the radio when you hear your favorite song.

I have asked several clients what they feel when I talk about acting without thinking, trusting on a deeper level. Here is what some of them said:

"Horrible."

"I cannot act without thinking, because I might make the wrong decision."

"It is scary—it could be a mistake, and then what would I do?"

BEING FULFILLED

"It is scary to make a mistake and then have to explain to people and myself why it was good at the time or why I was such an idiot."

"I would want to, but I won't."

"If I trust in someone else, then I cannot control the situation... what if they don't live up to my expectations and I get hurt?"

Most people have the idea that thinking through a situation will give them more control and things will work out the way they want them to. This goes back to wanting everything to be 100% perfect and therefore not having to change. When a situation does not work out the way you want it to, do you beat yourself up inside? Because often this is the case, people use logic so there is seemingly less pressure on themselves. They can then blame the external statistics, advice, and facts that they used to form their decision versus the internal gut feeling they initially had.

When you listen to your logic and fall short, you wind up saying things like, "If I had only..." or "I will never listen to that person or statistic again." When you listen to your heart and fall short, ideally you can be satisfied with the fact that you did all you could and followed your heart.

Think of how it feels when you get to the bottom of the barrel and say, "Screw it all!" Go to a time where you stopped caring what you and others thought and began acting from a place of passion. You gave yourself permission to be yourself and honored how you work. This is where you change the situation to fit you versus changing you to fit the situation.

Leap and the net will appear. How does that sound... scary or exhilarating? Being fulfilled is leaping and landing in that net. Frustration and the status quo are procrastination and complaining at the top. People who have leaped found out that the net was already there, but because their thinking clouded their vision, they could not see the net. How will it feel when you act before you think? The following is a real-life example of acting without thinking that my client sent me via email.

Client:

"Every now and then I run into an attractive man at the coffee shop that I stop at on my way to work. We run into each other two or three times a week. I have wanted to talk to him forever, but I keep thinking too much and scare myself out of doing so.

Today he was behind me in line while I was checking out. There were no other people in the shop, and I was feeling daring after all our coaching on being in the moment and acting from passion. When I paid for my coffee, I gave the girl extra money and left her my business card. I told her that I would like to buy his coffee and asked her to give him my card so he would have my name and number... I smiled at her and winked. She took the money and my card and nodded with an approving smile. Maybe nothing will come of it, but I felt great doing it, and I cannot wait till I bump into him again!"

BEING FULFILLED
What's Next?

In the first two sections we presented a new model for being fulfilled with ten solid philosophies and a seven-stage process for attaining it. The next three sections will utilize these seven stages by applying them to each of the three categories in our new model: business, relationship, and health.

Simply read each section first without doing the steps and exercises to begin to see how the seven stages are applied and where each of the philosophies fit. Because you can only focus on ONE area to create unlimited wealth, after you read all the sections, determine which of the three categories is your main focus: business, relationship, or health. Once you do that, reread that particular section and actively perform all the steps and exercises.

SECTION III

THE SEVEN STAGES APPLIED TO BUSINESS

How to Achieve Unlimited Wealth via Business

Once you have determined that business is the main focus in your life right now, invest some time and go through this section. Remember that when you focus on one area, in this case business, most of your energy and most of your time deserves to be there.

Now that you know unlimited wealth means complete fulfillment, it's important to ask yourself some pointed questions so you know exactly how to achieve this in your business.

Define business fulfillment as specifically as possible:_____

_____

_____

_____

BEING FULFILLED

Take a good look at your definition and revisit it often. As you continue to learn and grow, your definition will change. If you had trouble answering this question, you are not alone. Most people never take the time to define what they are doing, and therefore they lose focus. Some clients wrote that business fulfillment was having a lot of money. Know this: when you don't have the money, it is all about the money, but once you have the money, anyone will tell you that fulfillment in business becomes about something else.

The following are some questions that you can apply to your business. After these questions we will revisit the Seven Stages to Achieving Unlimited Wealth that you read about in the previous section. Once you go through the Seven Stages, come back and answer these questions. They are here to assist you in identifying what you are already clear on and what is a bit foggier. The Seven Stages will assist you in clarifying those foggy areas.

- *Define business success as specifically as possible.*
- *How will you know when you can slow down or stop your business?*
- *What is your big vision for your business?*
- *How clear is that big vision?*
- *How well does that vision keep you focused?*
- *How well do you focus?*
- *What is your purpose in business?*
- *What is the driving motivator that keeps you going every day?*
- *How is that motivator doing in achieving the results you desire?*
- *Define business results as specifically as possible.*

• *How well do you work alone?*

• *How organized are you?*

• *How are you when it comes to prioritizing business tasks?*

• *Describe the structure of your business day.*

• *How effective is the structure of your business day?*

• *What are the main strengths you possess in business?*

• *What are the areas you could be better at?*

• *What areas do you require of yourself to be better at?*

• *How well have you mastered the art of asking?*

• *How well have you mastered the art of following up?*

• *How do you manage stress?*

• *What happens to your mind (thoughts) and body (physical reactions) when you experience these emotions: frustration, anger, doubt, guilt, feeling overwhelmed, and anxiety?*

• *How do you deal with procrastination?*

• *Why do you procrastinate?*

• *How do you deal with success?*

• *How do you deal with failure?*

• *Would you do business with yourself? Why or why not?*

• *If someone were to watch you for a week while you work your business, what would they see?*

• *How would they describe your days?*

• *What are some gold nuggets that you do that they would want to duplicate in their business?*

• *What are some things you do that they would not what to duplicate?*

The Seven Stages to Achieve Unlimited Wealth via Business

Stage 1:
Create a Business Vision

Business provides you with the ability to further enjoy the other areas of your life by producing income security. This security allows you to do the things you want to do, when you want to do them, without fear or worry that there is not enough. In an ideal situation, your business is a place where you can harness your passions, skills, education, and creativity into a service or product that bears great value in the marketplace which you can exchange for large quantities of money.

You are not your business and your business is not you. Business is simply an entity in your life that provides different things at different times. If you rely on your business to provide too much, then it will almost always disappoint you. If you rely on your business for your identity, or if your business is a distraction from the rest of your life, then you are heading down the wrong road.

You must understand what your business is and how it fits into the rest of your life, just like everything else, it has a place. Most business people attempt to fit the rest of their life into their business... and that does not work in achieving unlimited wealth. There are appropriate times for doing business and others that are not appropriate. You must recognize these times if you desire fulfillment.

This is where creating a vision assists you greatly in business fulfillment. The only way you will create massive results, by your definition, in business is by creating a vision that is clear and certain. This vision allows you to see the path of how "it" will all play out in the future. "It" refers to your dreams and goals. This clear vision brings you to a place of certainty and belief, because now you can see all of these goals manifesting in reality.

When you truly see this clearly, you will feel like your results are no longer a matter of *if* they will happen but a matter of *when* they will happen. The powerful part now is that the *when* does not matter, because through this clear and certain vision, you know absolutely that it will happen. This is the situation we spoke of earlier: 0% Doubt = 100% Trust.

When you know deep inside that you will become a millionaire, the focus on becoming one and the anxiety around not being there yet goes away. Your vision gets rid of your fear, doubt, and overwhelmed feelings and grounds you so you have the ability to focus on the matter at hand. When there is no business vision, you have nothing to focus on, and therefore you float in procrastination.

BEING FULFILLED

How to Create a Clear and Certain Business Vision

A clear and certain vision typically is not created overnight. It can be done, but most likely it will not. In the world of business, the "how tos" of success can overwhelm the best of us. One of the easiest and best ways to create a business vision is a three-step process.

> *1) Find a person who is:*
>> *a) Doing what you want to do*
>> *b) Earning what you want to earn*
> *2) Model that person by mentoring, coaching, collaborating, and investing as much of your resources in learning how they do it. Understanding their model should provide a vision.*
> *3) Once you see your vision via their model, create your own model to achieve your vision.*

As you invest your time with these people from step one, you will quickly learn the habits and behaviors necessary to produce what they are producing. In order to grow anything, you must become someone who deserves that result. The more you surround yourself with these people and learn what they have to teach you, you can then begin to formulate your own vision.

Begin to apply what they do to your own business, and be sure you recognize that modeling is not copying. Your model must be your own, not someone else's. **Modeling allows you to see your potential and your vision in their model. Once you see your potential, you can create your own model to achieve your vision.**

Example

As we go through these seven stages, let's use Steve as an example of how each stage is applied. Steve is a middle-aged father of one and has been happily married for several years. He takes great care of his health and has for many years. He is very close to his two siblings and his parents. Steve loves to play sports, and he has several other hobbies that he loves. He is a proud father and has a dog that he loves as well. Steve has several close friends that he loves to see and spend time with. He has several jobs, and for the past several years he also has been trying to grow his own business as a speaker. Financially he earns enough to pay the bills—but not without worry. He has invested in the stock market for several years and has a decent portfolio.

Steve knows that he has the potential to be wildly successful and can envision this success. His visions however have not been at a level that releases his anxiety and worries. As an entrepreneur who has a new idea every day and a million other things to do, he tends to just struggle, remain the same, and not accomplish much. Steve knew he needed to create a clearer and more certain vision for his speaking business, so he used the three steps we just presented.

1) Find a person who is:
      a) Doing what you want to do
      b) Earning what you want to earn

It took Steve about a year before he found the right person. He began going to different seminars and calling different speakers he knew to learn more about their business. He hired them as coaches and mentored with several of them, but he did not find much connection with what he was passionate about for *his* business. After looking into and learning about several seminar companies and speakers, Steve finally came across a speaker who he saw himself in. "This speaker is doing exactly what I want to do and is earning more than I could even dream of!" Steve thought. At this point, Steve knew he had completed step one and began step two.

2) Model that person by mentoring, coaching, collaborating, and investing as much of your resources into learning how they do it.

Steve immediately hired this speaker as his coach and mentor so he could begin to learn how his business worked. Steve went to his events, read his books, listened to his recordings, and did everything his coach told him to. Steve even had the opportunity to collaborate with this speaker and do a few events together. That was exciting!

One day, Steve had a vividly clear vision of how he would succeed as a speaker. He began to see specifically how his business would look ten, twenty, and even thirty years down the road. He now convincingly saw how he could easily be a multiple six- and even seven-figure income earner, even though at the time he could barely pay the next month's mortgage.

Steve was able to see this because he clearly learned how someone else was doing it. He then had the vision of how he specifically could do the same thing, but in his own way. Even though he was not there yet and realized it would take many years to get there, this clear vision of "how to" instantly released the pressure to do it now along with the anxiety of results not happening quickly enough. This vision also showed him exactly what the next big step was in his own speaking business and essentially planned out his day-to-day actions. Steve moved on to step three:

3) Once you to see your vision via their model, create your own model to achieve your vision.

Week by week, Steve began creating his own model based on this clear vision he had. He easily began to recognize all the "stuff" in his day that was slowing him down. He felt very excited and yet relaxed because he now had the certainty inside that he was going to make it. Steve recognized that the model that he was creating was going to take time. He knew it would evolve as time passed and as he learned more. He was okay with that because the big vision kept him grounded, and he discovered that being grounded was the only way he could create consistent, bold action.

Stage 2:
Simplify and Prioritize from that Vision

When your business vision is super clear and certain inside, the need for this second stage will be very obvious. One thing to remember about these seven stages is that going through them should feel natural and effortless. In other words, once you complete a stage, the next stage should seem very appropriate and necessary. How appropriate and necessary depends on the degree of clarity and certainty of your vision.

Your clear business vision is like putting on a special pair of glasses that point out all the activities and commitments in your life that distract you from succeeding. Activities that produce results in business are called "revenue-producing activities." Activities that produce results in life are called "results-producing activities." The simplification process of Stage Two is designed to rid your time in business and life of activities that keep you busy and direct you towards revenue-producing and results-producing activities that keep you focused. Remember Philosophy#9: Become Focused, Not Busy.

It is imperative to point out that when you simplify, you must look at all your commitments. There are two types of commitments: physical and emotional. A physical commitment might be helping a friend move. This requires you to be physically present and uses physical time and energy. An emotional commitment might be volunteering to have a holiday get-together over your house versus simply going to someone else's. When you do something like that, there is a lot of emotional planning and energy focused around preparing for the get-together, much of which is not physical.

This "emotional contract" can stress different people out at different levels just by thinking about the occasion. This emotional type of commitment is more draining than most of us realize. This is why it is so important you understand that you only have ten energy points each day. If most of your points, most of the time, are to be invested in your business, any physical and emotional commitments that distract you from this focus **must be deleted** from your day.

Once you have identified the areas that deserve to go and the ones that deserve to stay, prioritizing these activities is a must. You may not know exactly what all these activities are yet, so this is why it is important to work closely with a coach or mentor who can assist you in discovering what works for you.

Seven Steps on How to Simplify and Prioritize from Your Business Vision

1) Create a list of all the activities/commitments you do in a typical week broken down by each day.

2) Estimate how many of your ten energy points each activity takes. Overestimate, because they will use more than you want or think they will!

3) Determine how appropriate each activity is in relation to the success of your business vision.

4) Decide which activities need to go completely or be cut back.

5) With the activities you have left, go back to step one and repeat this process two more times!

6) Prioritize your remaining activities/commitments with a ranking of one, two, and three. One is the most revenue/ results producing and three is the least. The more you simplify, the more everything will seem like a one. This is how you know you have done a great job of simplifying. Add to this the very important activities that you are not doing but know are required, and rank them as well.

7) Communicate necessary changes with the appropriate people. Set your boundaries!

Example

Steve was thrilled about the momentum that his clear vision created in his business. As he was in the process of creating his business model, knowing clearly all the actions he needed to take to succeed, he became very overwhelmed. He felt overwhelmed, because with all the commitments in his life—all the things he had to do, wanted to do, and needed to do—he did not have the time or the energy to do it all. This is where he knew Stage Two was very much needed.

Steve ran himself through the seven steps to simplify and prioritize from his vision, and here is what he came up with.

1) Create a list of all the activities/commitments you do in a typical week broken down by each day.

2) Estimate how many of your ten energy points each activity takes.

Let's take a look at two typical days in the life of Steve:

	Average Day 1	Energy Pts.	Average Day 2	Energy Pts.
6:00 AM 7:00 AM	Get up, clean up, read paper, eat, check email	2	Get up, clean up, vacuum house, eat, Clean, and organize	4
8:00 AM	Be a dad, multitask, household duties, make a few calls	4	Be a dad, multitask, household duties	4
9:00 AM 10:00 AM 11:00 AM	Commute time, workout at gym Do an errand or two	4	Commute time, do an errand	
12:00 PM 1:00 PM 2:00 PM 3:00 PM 4:00 PM	Commute time, do an errand Work at one of his draining part-time jobs Check email, Make a few calls, Commute time	7	Work at one of his draining part-time jobs Check email, make a few calls Commute time	12
5:00 PM 6:00 PM	Go home and work On his speaking business	3	Be a dad and husband, do errands, eat, call friends	4
7:00 PM 8:00 PM	Be a dad and husband, make dinner, clean house, eat	4	Commute time Workout at gym, go shopping on way home	4
9:00 PM	Watch TV, relax, be a husband	2	Commute time, hang out with friends make dinner while on phone, eat	3
10:00 PM	Check email, surf Internet	2	Check email, work on speaking business	3
	Total Energy Points	28	Total Energy Points	34

After creating this chart, it was clear to Steve why he had no time to do everything, and why he was not successful in his business. The rest of his days looked even worse. On top of all this, he noticed how high his energy points were each day… and he felt it, too! He was not surprised to see that virtually none of his activities were revenue or results producing. Even his workouts at the gym were mediocre nowadays. This is when he proceeded to step three.

> 3) *Determine how appropriate each activity is in relation to the success of your business vision.*

This was easy for Steve, because so much of his time was spent just getting by. There were only a few times in a day where he honestly had some productive time in the different parts of his life. He proceeded...

> 4) *Decide which activities need to go completely or be cut back.*
> 5) *With the activities you have left, go back to step one and repeat this process two more times!*

Steve originally thought the part of deleting and cutting back on activities would be the most difficult, but it was not. This confirmed that his business vision was clear. Here are some of the weekly activities that Steve cut out completely (some seen on the chart and some not): Watching television, aimlessly surfing the Internet and checking email, reading the paper, and a few of his hobbies.

The biggest decision that was evident to Steve was that he had to quit his jobs! Even though he was struggling to pay the bills and did not yet have much income from his speaking business, it was clear that until he stopped these jobs, it would be nearly impossible to be successful in his own business. Steve was surprised how comfortable he was in this decision to quit, because in the past he never thought he could. This is another testament to what a powerful vision can do.

Steve continued through the first four steps a few more times. He cut down on time spent with friends and outside family members, and he also cut back several of his workouts each week, while increasing their quality.

> *6) Prioritize remaining activities/commitments with a ranking of one, two, and three. Add activities you know are required but are not doing.*
>
> *7) Communicate necessary changes with the appropriate people. Set your boundaries!*

Because of his clear vision, Steve was able to quit his jobs and weed out his commitments by applying the ten key philosophies outlined in the previous section. Yes, he had some rough days and some second-guesses, but in the end his vision kept him moving forward. With all the free time Steve created, he saw the importance of prioritizing his remaining activities with the ones he wanted to add. He knew it was important to keep the fluff out and only add result-producing activities.

Not only did Steve rank his most important activities, but he also had necessary conversations with his friends, family, and wife to communicate what he was doing. He had to set his boundaries clearly, so he would not feel guilty or like he was neglecting the important people in his life. He had done this in the past without the communication part, and the guilt and outside pressure from other people zapped his energy.

Stage 3:
Structure and Organize Your Days around Your Priorities

Structure is the main ingredient to any success story. No matter who you are, if your days just happen and you don't know what you are doing next, you will fail... end of story. If you are busy all day but not organized with systems and processes, your results will be mediocre at best. Most people who have their own business keep themselves busy with paperwork, learning, personal development, and distracting to dos, all which in the end get them nowhere.

Most entrepreneurs who have a job in addition to their business want to quit so badly. They desire free time to do what they want, when they want. They not only romance the idea of earning more money, but they also have the impression that they can work whenever they want to, set their own hours... essentially have no structure. The ones that actually become full-time entrepreneurs love the time freedom for the first few weeks—at least until they run out of money and the bills keep coming in. What many entrepreneurs do not realize is that being successful in your own business begins with two things:

1) You must treat your business just like a job!

You must have office hours, filing systems, follow-up systems, an organized database, information that is easily and quickly located and accessible, and a clean and neat environment conducive to producing results. You must show up each and every day for a full day's work at least five days a week. You even need a consistent wake-up time and bedtime each day to stay on schedule.

The main difference is that in a job, if you don't produce results or show up, you run the risk of getting fired. This can keep a person on schedule and producing. As an entrepreneur, no one is watching you and holding you accountable. So if you don't show up or produce, you will just be broke... and for the average person, being broke does not seem like a big enough motivator.

2) Your business deserves to be full-time

There are people that can become largely successful doing a business part-time... whatever part-time means for you. In reality, you (**yes, you**) statistically will accomplish beige results at best in anything if you remain part-time. If you feel like you are putting in full-time hours and full-time energy but are still getting mediocre results, have a coach or a mentor take a look at what you are really doing. Share your activities with other highly successful people to determine what is necessary to change.

In this stage, we bring up the concept of having uncompromisable time. This is time where under any circumstances besides an extreme emergency, you DO NOT COMPROMISE. This time is especially important for items outside your focus area so you don't feel like you are neglecting them. Ensuring that your structure includes only revenue- and results-producing activities is very important. It might at times feel like hard sacrifice and discipline not having some activities you consider to be "fun" or "relaxing"; however, your vision should allow you to clearly see that your sacrifices will not have to be forever once you produce the type of results you are going after in your business.

BEING FULFILLED

The new structure that you will create will allow you to finish your days before you start them. This means you will clearly see the end of your day and all that you will produce via your scheduled actions. This allows you to move through your day with a lot less effort and ease and allows your ten energy points to go further than they previously did.

Six Steps to Structure and Organize Your Day

1) Determine your wake-up time and bedtime each day.

2) Determine your office hours each day. Too many frequent breaks will cause you to lose focus and not be able to create any momentum. A three-hour block is a minimum recommendation for business hours.

3) Determine your revenue-producing activities and where they should go during your business hours.

4) Determine your results-producing activities outside your business and schedule uncompromisable time for those activities.

5) Take a close look at your organizational systems in and out of your business and begin to improve their effectiveness.

6) Stick to your new structure for a minimum of three months.

Example

Because Steve deleted and cut back on many activities, at first it seemed like he almost had too much time on his hands. He knew that when this happened in the past, he would fill time with useless activities to keep himself from being bored. Before he structured his days, he would spend lots of time doing nothing, just keeping busy. He quickly recognized the importance of having a clear structure and more organization. He actually found that once he structured his day, he accomplished more in less time with less energy.

He was much more flexible because of all this freedom he had created; there were no pressure or deadlines like he had in his job. Steve used the flexibility of his new schedule to create uncompromisable time for his results-producing activities. Because his old schedule was so hectic and inflexible, he could never find a specific time to do anything and keep it there. Now with his flexible schedule, he was better able to schedule that uncompromisable time where it was most effective. Take a look at Steve's simplified, structured schedule.

	New Day 1	Energy Pts.	New Day 2	Energy Pts.
6:00 AM	Get up, clean up		Get up, clean up	
7:00 AM		1		1
	Be a dad, eat with son		Be a dad, eat with son	
8:00 AM				
9:00 AM				
10:00 AM				
11:00 AM				
12:00 PM	Work on his speaking business	6	Work on his speaking business	5
1:00 PM				
2:00 PM				
3:00 PM				
4:00 PM			Go to gym and workout	2
5:00 PM				
6:00 PM	Be a dad and husband, eat with family	1	Be a dad and husband, eat with family	1
7:00 PM				
8:00 PM				
9:00 PM	Work on his speaking business	2	Work on his speaking business	1
10:00 PM				
	Total Energy Points	10	Total Energy Points	10

As you can see, he removed a lot of activities. Best of all, his total energy points each day came to ten… and he could feel the difference. Because he was so relaxed and present in each of his scheduled activities, he found himself using lots less energy to produce a greater result. As oppose to doing a million other things (multitasking) in the morning with his son, he was simply with his son. Instead of wasting time in front of the television and other mindless activities, he was easily able to fit in the important activities and devote more quality time to each. After creating this schedule, Steve ran himself through the six steps to structure and organize his day.

1) Determine your wake-up time and bedtime each day

In the past this would vary, depending on many things. Steve knew that he thrived on seven to eight hours of sleep each night. Because his son got up between 6:30-7:00 a.m. consistently, he decided to get up at 6:00 a.m. to ensure that he would have time to take care of himself and any other miscellaneous items before his son woke up. This allowed Steve to just be with his son and not have to multitask. With that wake-up time being clear, it was easy for Steve to decide on a bedtime of 10:30 p.m. These hours gave him plenty of time to accomplish what was required of him, because he weeded out so many nonessential activities.

2) Determine your office hours each day.
3) Determine your revenue-producing activities and where they should go during your business hours.

Steve knew it was imperative to treat his business like a full-time job if he wanted to produce a full-time paycheck. He also knew that because his habits and some necessary skills were not as good as he would like them to be, he would require more than just a typical forty-hour work week. He determined that it was necessary to work Monday through Friday from 9:00 a.m. to 5:00 p.m., with one of those days finishing at 4:00 p.m. To get in some bonus hours in his business, he included a few blocks of time in the evening after his wife and son went to bed.

BEING FULFILLED

Now that his business hours were set, Steve had to ensure he was not just pushing papers all day. This is where Steve used many of the ten key philosophies outlined earlier to assist him in producing more with less effort. He took a look at what his coach and mentor did on a daily basis to produce results, and he then performed those actions within his own business model.

Because the nature of his business was fairly unpredictable and he did not have much to schedule during his business day, it was even more important to keep certain times during his business day for uncompromisable activities like prospecting, following up, setting up seminars, closing clients, and effective marketing. These were major revenue-producing activities that he could not afford to compromise. Now that he had his business day figured out for the time being, he moved on to the next step.

> 4) *Determine your results-producing activities outside your business and schedule uncompromisable time for those activities.*

Because Steve cared dearly about his wife, son, and dog, he did not want to compromise his relationship with them. He also valued his health, and he had worked on it for so long that he could not let that go downhill. Because most of his energy most of the time was devoted to his business, he had to make sure that the other two components of his life stayed connected if he wanted to create unlimited wealth.

Uncompromisable Relationship Time

He determined that results-producing activities in his relationship consisted of at least one solid block of time each day where he could fully concentrate on his son and wife, either as individuals or as a family. He communicated his focus clearly and effectively to his wife, and she did the same with hers. They determined as a team that he would be responsible for being a dad when their son woke up until his workday began each day at 9:00 a.m. This would give Steve's wife a solid four hours each morning to focus on herself, since she was an early riser. This chunk of time each morning allowed Steve to simply be a dad and focus on his son.

This morning time was uncompromisable time with his son. Steve created the new habit that, no matter what opportunity he had, he would not compromise or trade his time with his son. The only exception to this rule was an obvious emergency or an insane opportunity that nobody in their right mind could pass up. Because Steve set up this uncompromisable time, he didn't feel like he was neglecting his son, which allowed him to better focus on producing during his business day.

Steve and his wife recognized the importance of being a family and having alone time as a couple, too. They selected two of the five weekdays from 5:00 p.m. to 8:00 p.m. to stop all other aspects of life and just be a family. They actually scheduled time to cook a meal together and sit at the table and eat like a real family. Once dinner was complete, they would all clean up together, play a little, and do the nighttime rituals they wanted to implement. They realized that if their son thrived off a strict schedule, it would only make sense if they did too.

When it came to alone time as a couple, Steve and his wife determined that at least once a month they would find a babysitter so they could go out alone during that 5:00 p.m. to 8:00 p.m. time frame. **This "family time" was uncompromisable time.** Steve and his wife created the habit that, no matter what came up, they would honor this time. They only way they could change this time would be to have a discussion and both agree it was necessary to change it. They both agreed that the reason would have to be very important if they were to compromise this "family time."

Uncompromisable Health Time

Steve was in great shape and worked out regularly, so allowing his health to slide was not an option for him. Even though he valued his health very much, he recognized that continuing his rigorous workout and athletic schedule cut too much into his business focus and uncompromisable family time. Steve came to terms with the fact that he deserved to find the least amount of workout time possible for him to maintain his level of physical and emotional health without letting it slide.

When Steve added up all his exercise time, he discovered that he was investing nine hours each week working out. He chose his three best workouts, shortened the duration, and ramped up the intensity of each. This created an extra five hours each week that he strategically placed into his new structure. He was able to expand his office hours and keep his family time. **These three workouts were Steve's uncompromisable health time.**

The key to Steve's success was that he carved out specific times each week for his uncompromisable relationship and health time. He did not rely on just trying to fit it in whenever. He scheduled the same times each week, and he did not veer from that schedule. At first it was hard, because he was not used to it. But after only a few weeks, he began to rely on the new schedule, and he actually felt that he was getting more from each of his ten energy points. Steve proceeded to the next step.

5) Take a close look at your organizational systems in and out of your business and begin to improve their effectiveness.

Even though Steve scheduled uncompromisable time in all three categories of business, relationships, and heath, his organizational skills had a lot of flaws. He had no systems and processes for any of the three areas. He would waste minutes at a time searching for papers in his office, he would lose valuable time with his son and wife because the everyday household duties were not getting done, and his now shortened workouts were still not effective because he had no plan. Step five allowed him to:

1) Create necessary systems and processes in his business to save time and energy

2) Establish who does what, when, and how in the house and relationship

3) Systemize his workouts precisely to get in and out with zero wasted time and still achieve a killer workout.

Like any new endeavor, things rarely work flawlessly the first time... or the second or third! Steve and his wife missed family time more than once. Steve would carelessly schedule a networking meeting for 7:30-9:00 a.m., compromising time with his son. He would have trouble fitting a client in, so he would prostitute his exercise time just to fit the client in so he could make a buck. Steve quickly discovered that this did not work. Uncompromisable does not mean flexible. Steve had a conversation with his wife and one with his coach, and it became clear that if he wanted to be fulfilled, he deserved to stick to his new structure. Then came step six.

> *6) Stick to your new structure for a minimum of three months.*

At first Steve felt this new structure, organization, and rules were suffocating and restricting. He felt a lack of freedom, which was what he was looking for as an entrepreneur. When these feelings became too much, Steve was tempted to add some flexibility to his week. But every time he veered from the schedule, it seemed like his whole world fell out of whack, and his energy would deplete very quickly. Through coaching, he learned that he was not the only person who felt this way. He logically knew the benefits of structure and scheduling, but he had not truly experienced the benefits of them yet.

As an entrepreneur, you cannot rely on logical knowledge to keep you in the game. **You just have to stay in the game long enough to experience the results.** There is no easy way to put it. If your vision is clear enough, it will allow you the focus to keep at your new structure. This is why you must stick to your new structure for a minimum of three months. If you keep changing things around, you will never get good at them, you'll never adapt, and you'll be constantly wasting precious energy points adapting to a new environment.

Steve found that the longer he stuck with his new structure, the easier it became and ironically, the more freeing it felt. At first it felt restrictive, because he "had to" do a certain activity at a specific time. Over time, however, he experienced relief that he did not have to worry about when he would work out, see his wife, spend time with his son, or have adequate time to produce results in his business. Because of his predictable schedule, he knew exactly when he would fit his activities in, and he rested easier because of that.

Stage 4:
Know Yourself and Establish Your New Rules

Now that you have simplified and prioritized from your vision and have created a structure around it, it's necessary to understand how you perform in this new environment. This stage is dedicated to discovering how you operate under all conditions — daytime, nighttime, stressful times, abundant times, poverty times, healthy times, unhealthy times, and any condition you can imagine.

After graduation, a college friend of mine became a fighter pilot in the air force, just like Tom Cruise in the movie *Top Gun*. Before he could even step into a real fighter jet, though, he had to go through training eight hours a day for over a year and a half. The school simulated every condition known to man to see how the potential pilots would perform. Daytime, nighttime, sleet, fog, rain, sun, snow, malfunctions, etc. — they had to know what every button did under every condition. They had to understand themselves and how they responded to these conditions.

You are no different in your environment, especially since your brain has a billion more functions and capabilities than a fighter jet. If you don't know how you operate under even the calmest conditions, you will crash and burn. Realize that the odds are not in your favor to succeed; they are not in anyone's favor, so you'd be wise to create better odds by learning your equipment.

BEING FULFILLED

Once you begin to learn to know yourself better, you must create new rules that serve you. Philosophy #10, Act Before You Think, will assist you with this. Here you challenge all your rules in the game of business to see what creates results and what resists results. You begin to look at the values you possess and leverage your results through those values and ethics.

Leveraging Your Values in Business

A client, Jennifer, was constantly late for everything. Whether it was showing up for work, a family get-together, delivering a promised document, or a phone appointment... Jennifer was habitually late. Everyone in her world came to expect that she would be late. It was her mojo, as she called it.

She had wanted to start her own business for a while. Recognizing that she had no time and energy to do it with her current job, she quit! As she began her entrepreneurial journey, she found that being late in her own business is not good for business. Her big problem: she was habitually late. No matter how hard she tried, she was still late. In fact, the harder she tried to be on time, the later she was!

Through coaching, we discovered two values that she held very important in her life:

1) Respect for other people's time
2) Keeping her word

Especially now with her own business, she found that being late and breaking promises to clients were in direct conflict with those two values. It was evident that trying hard was not working to change this habit, so this is where we brought her values into play. (The idea is to leverage your values to essentially force you to do what you want to do and not feel like it is an effort. It's finding a way to put your values on the line with a hefty risk on the other end so they propel you into the desired result.)

Here's what Jennifer did. She drafted a letter she called her "On Time Guarantee." This was a contract that she would give to a new or prospective client which stated that for the life of their business relationship she would guarantee timeliness on all appointments, phone calls, and deliverables within five minutes of the agreed upon time. If for *whatever reason* she was more than five minutes late (this accounted for discrepancies in clocks), she would write a check for $500 and give it to the client... no questions asked, no excuses good enough!

Jennifer put her values on the line, which she wanted to honor so badly, and she created a situation where it would cost her dearly if she did not honor them. Jennifer did not have money to spare, so $500 was a massive hit to her bank account. Jennifer leveraged her values with money as a risk to ensure her success. As soon as she implemented this, she was instantly five to ten minutes early for everything! The best part is that she did not even feel as if she had to try to be early—it was automatic.

In order for this to work, she had to share this with everyone, and she had to follow through. Not only did this contract work for her goals, but it also added a valuable component to her business. Jennifer sold insurance and like she said, "Everyone sells insurance!" This "On Time Guarantee" separated her from her competitors, especially since the industry is not very predictable. Guaranteeing her promises and always being on time added huge value to her business and allowed her to increase profits almost immediately.

In order for this to work, she had to share this with everyone, and she had to follow through. Not only did this contract work for her goals, but it also added a valuable component to her business. Jennifer sold insurance and like she said, "Everyone sells insurance!" This "On Time Guarantee" separated her from her competitors, especially since the industry is not very predictable. Guaranteeing her promises and always being on time added huge value to her business and allowed her to increase profits almost immediately.

As of this writing, Jennifer has been doing her "On Time Guarantee" for five months, and it is working flawlessly. She *did* have to pay one client the $500 due to getting caught in a traffic jam. Jennifer did not make excuses, she paid the reward, and she now has a client for life—a great testimonial that she follows through with her word, and above all, a system that works!

Three Steps to Understand Yourself, Your Rules… and Change!

1) Create an Awareness of Current Behaviors
2) Identify Triggers and Current Rules
3) Consciously Practice New Responses

Here you create an awareness of what is keeping you doing the same thing over and over again. You identify the triggers and rules that set your old behavior patterns in motion. Then you break those old patterns by practicing new responses and creating a new rule book. You create rules that serve you versus hold you back. You challenge everything you know to see how it fits into your new focus.

Example

Now that Steve's schedule was set and he was sticking to it, he noticed other problems. Even though he had a clear vision, focused time, and was more relaxed, he did not know how to act when "life" got in the way. Just because he had a set schedule and had communicated clearly to everyone, it was not always calm seas ahead. Steve began to notice that his life had many different conditions within the structure he had created. It was his job to maintain this structure, but these external conditions, those he could not control, kept getting in the way.

What happened when he, his son, or his wife was sick? How did he react when he did not close a speaking engagement or client? What about when he did? He noticed that when he was frustrated, disappointed, or overwhelmed, it would still paralyze him for days, or even weeks. Sometimes his family or friends would have a get-together during his business day or his uncompromisable times. Even though Steve had communicated his boundaries to these people, they still seemed to lay a guilt trip on him or tried to persuade him to change his schedule. Steve thought that having a structure would have cured all this, but it did not.

Steve was a great student, so he knew he could not change his external environment and the people in it. He recognized the importance of this stage, where he began to understand himself and create new rules that would work for him. He now saw all his disempowering emotions and situations as opportunities to learn more about how he acted so he could respond favorably in the future. He knew this would allow him to produce more results with less energy.

Understand Yourself—Emotions

Like most people, Steve did not have a handle on his emotions. He used the three steps just presented to focus his emotions.

1) Create an Awareness of Current Behaviors

Steve had a tough time structuring his mindset to match the schedule of his day. In other words, when Steve was working his business, his mind was telling him he should be playing with his son. When he was playing with his son, he was thinking about all the work he had to do. *He had the physical structure in place, but not the mental structure.* One of the emotions that took Steve out of the game way too often was guilt.

Steve valued many things, and too often these values came in conflict with each other. Even though his schedule said one thing, many times he was not mentally present for that one thing. An example was when he was working in his home office. Many times he would hear his son crying for long periods of time. He knew that his wife was taking care of things, but he also knew she was tired. In addition, he knew how frustrating it was when his son cried and he and his wife didn't know what to do. Steve would sit in his office feeling guilty for not helping her. Meanwhile, he was not doing anything productive in his business.

This happened day after day. When his business day was over and it was time to be with his son, Steve would feel guilty once again because he had not accomplished anything in his business that day. Steve followed the structure of his day, but he did not understand his emotions well enough to match the structure with his mindset. Steve was very aware of this, and he knew it had to stop.

2) Identify Triggers

Each of Steve's emotions had different triggers. In this particular example, his baby crying triggered guilt. Through coaching, Steve discovered that guilt was simply a conflict between two values that cannot be honored at the same time. He valued being a great dad, yet he also valued his business. Guilt came into play because he could not honor both values at the same time and still be productive.

3) Consciously Practice New Responses

Steve's new response when he heard his baby crying was to stop what he was doing in his office. He would acknowledge the feeling he was experiencing, in this case guilt. He would begin to coach himself by asking questions like: "What specific action would allow me to honor the value I've placed on my business, yet not feel like I am neglecting my other values?" One of his actions was to ask his wife if she was able to handle the situation. Steve cared deeply and wanted to help when he could. He reconfirmed to his wife that he needed to work and that they both were okay with their current roles.

This conversation essentially gave Steve permission to work and not feel guilty, because he knew his wife and son were fine, and he had honored that value. This communication worked great for Steve; he was able to get back to his office and produce for the rest of the day. This simple conversation took only five minutes, whereas before he would waste entire days feeling like this. Steve took the same three steps with his other emotions and was able to produce significant results.

Understand Yourself – New Rules

Now that Steve was well on his way to understanding his emotions, he began to apply the same three steps to understanding his current rules and learning how to create new ones.

SECTION III – THE SEVEN STAGES APPLIED TO BUSINESS

1) Create an Awareness of Current Behaviors
2) Identify Triggers and Current Rules

One rule that wasted a lot Steve's time was "Don't wait until the last minute to do things." In other words, if the deadline is in three months, start now so you are not pulling all-nighters and stressing out at the last minute. Even though Steve grew up hearing this from everyone, he still always waited to the last minute to do things. The worst part was that if a deadline was three months away, he would stress out the whole three months, thinking he should be doing something. This stress zapped his valuable energy points and resulted in decreased productivity. His triggers were everywhere, because he always had deadlines. This rule resulted in behavior that had to change.

3) Consciously Practice New Responses

Steve knew this rule might be appropriate for some but not for him. He challenged this by doing the opposite. He waited to the last possible moment on all deadlines during a three-month trial period to see if his results would change. If he had a project due in two weeks, he would simply go out two weeks in his calendar, a day or two before the due date, block off what he felt were enough hours, and then forget about the project. When the scheduled time arrived, he would use that allotted time to complete the project.

Steve found that not only would he get it done "last minute," he would do an incredible job... much better than if he tried to do it ahead of time. He discovered that he worked much more efficiently and was super productive when he had a time crunch and the pressure was on... as opposed to stressing for the whole two weeks because the deadline was getting closer and he was not doing anything.

This is a great example of how Steve began to understand how he worked. This process required Steve to trust his eye for quality and have faith that he would not do a half-assed job in the last minutes before the deadline. His ability to look at a rule objectively allowed him to use time stress as fuel versus as a brake. Steve frequently practiced Philosophy #5 to help him adopt his new rules: When You Judge Yourself Less and Trust More, You Will Have Everything You Want.

Stage 5:
Find the Right People to Maintain the Focus and Support the Vision

In this stage you realize that you cannot attain unlimited wealth alone. It does not matter what type of industry or business you are in—the path to unlimited riches, relationships, and health are through your network of people. It has been said that the person with the biggest Rolodex wins… and they would be correct. Who you are connected to and who assists you day-to-day is one of the biggest factors in your business fulfillment.

One of the greatest athletes of all time, Lance Armstrong, is a prime example of this. Lance was a young professional cyclist when he was terminally diagnosed with testicular, brain, and lung cancer. His doctor said he had no chance of survival, although he did not tell Lance that. Lance not only went on to beat cancer, but he returned to professional cycling and won what has been said to be the most grueling athletic event ever, the Tour de France.

The Tour de France is the world's best-known cycling race, a twenty-two day, twenty-stage road race that usually runs more than two thousand miles long through areas of France and its surrounding countries. Lance not only won this race, he won it seven times in a row! No other cyclist in the Tour de France's 104-year history has ever done this.

The only way Lance was able to achieve such an accomplishment was to align himself with the right people to maintain his focus and support his vision. Contrary to what people might think, at this level, cycling is first and foremost a team sport. The Tour de France consists of about twenty teams with nine riders on each team. Each team has its leader—the person they think can win. Because only one person can win the race, it is up to the rest of the team to ensure that their leader finishes first. These riders are called domestiques. They work solely for the benefit of their team leader. The French word *domestique* literally translates as "servant."

These domestiques have many roles during the twenty-two-day race. One of these roles is to create a slipstream that the leader can ride behind. This technique is termed "drafting" and is a key to conserving energy. For instance, if you were on a bike and your friend was riding in front of you, it would behoove you to stay as close to their back wheel as possible in a tucked down position. Essentially, they would be blocking all the oncoming wind and you would expend a lot less energy—roughly 40 percent less energy! But don't get the wrong impression that the domestiques do it all; the leader can absolutely pull his or her own weight. It just goes to show that no matter how great you are, you cannot do it alone.

Let's take a look at some of the other roles domestiques have in a cycling race:

   1) Basic Support

BEING FULFILLED

Some general tasks carried out by the domestiques include retrieving water and nutrition from the team cars and bringing it back to the rest of the team. They also shield their teammates from aggressive opponents. Domestiques are vital in helping teammates cope with mechanical disasters. Should the leader suffer a tire puncture, the domestique will shield them as they pull over, wait with them until they have replaced the tire, and then cycle in front of them to create a draft that pulls the leader back into the race, quickly allowing them to reclaim their position. A domestique may also be called upon to sacrifice his or her bicycle if necessary.

2) Tactical Support

Domestiques are also important for racing in a way that is in the tactical interest of their own team, one that is against the tactical interest of opposing teams. Let's say Lance Armstrong is in the lead, and it's getting close to the last day of the race. There are several other teams in contention who could easily steal the victory from Lance. If the domestiques from a contending team decide to break away from the main field, Lance and his team have no choice but to keep pace and stay ahead of them, or he might lose the race.

Domestiques will also help sprinters by giving them a "lead out." The domestique will race at a high tempo with the sprinter drafting behind and conserving energy until the last few hundred meters. The sprinter will then launch himself from behind the draft, hopefully across the finish line. Similarly, the domestiques that are better climbers will help their team leader by setting a pace up the big climbs, making sure their opponents don't get too far ahead.

3) Hierarchy among Domestiques

There is a hierarchy among domestiques. The more accomplished riders are called "lieutenants." These riders are called upon especially during critical times in a race. Generally, the lieutenants will stay with the team leader as long as possible during this demanding time. Lance Armstrong typically used two or three lieutenants to set a vicious pace during key mountain stages of the Tour de France, leaving his competitors crushed somewhere down the mountain because they could not keep up. One at a time, these lieutenants would burn out and drop off the back. When no one was left, Lance attacked his way to victory.

In addition to the domestiques, Lance had a team of trainers and coaches who kept him physically at the top of his game. He had specific eating regimens designed by a nutritionist and prepared by the team chef. He had a scientific team improving the equipment he used to ensure each and every detail assisted him with his vision of winning the Tour. For example, the people at Nike who engineered his body suit would look at the wind resistance of something as small as a seam. They would then redesign the seams to minimize the wind resistance.

Bottom line: nothing in life is an individual sport. Your business is no different than winning the Tour. If you try and do it alone, all the luck in the world will not help. Let's take a look at how Steve implemented the right people to maintain his focus and support his vision.

Example

As Steve's business grew, he noticed that even though his time was well structured and he was working efficiently, he was still not able to accomplish everything he wanted to, both in his business and in the other areas of his life. Stage Six was paramount for Steve to maintain what he had created and especially to take his business to the next level. Steve used the concept of the domestique and their "roles" to incorporate the right people into his world.

1) Basic Support

This basic support took place *outside* business. As Steve's income grew, he realized how valuable his time was. He knew that activities such as cleaning the house, grocery shopping, vacuuming, paying the bills, and simple errands like going to the bank, while necessary to do, were not results-producing activities; they pulled him away from his main focus. Steve also had invested lots of time with some very affluent business people, and they all agreed that without the right people, they never would have been able to be as profitable as they were.

Steve knew it was time to hire the right people to assist him with some basic support. He knew it would be an investment, and he did not quite "have the money" to hire these people. Steve revisited Philosophy #3: Fulfillment Is Not a Matter of Circumstance; It Is Largely a Matter of Conscious Choice. Steve knew his financial situation was a circumstance, and he would not let that get in the way.

Because his vision was so clear and certain, he did not worry like he had in the past about money. He clearly saw his riches and knew he was on the right path to attain them. He knew that *the money never comes first.* If he kept waiting to afford the right people, he would never earn more, because those people were necessary for him to earn it. **People come first; the money will follow.**

The first thing Steve did was look for a landscaper to take care of his property. Even though he enjoyed and took pride caring for his property, it had to go. That afforded him an extra three hours each week! The funny part was that it only cost him fifty dollars to gain that time by hiring that landscaper. Before long, he wondered why he hadn't done this sooner.

Steve and his wife also hired a nanny to assist them a few times each week. This not only freed up his wife to produce more money, but on her own the nanny also began to do some housecleaning when the baby was sleeping. Steve and his wife began to notice how clean their house was, and also how much extra time they had together because of this! They approached the nanny the next day and offered to pay her more for adding cleaning to her responsibilities. The nanny accepted, and Steve had even more time and energy to produce!

2) Tactical Support

Tactical support took place *inside* Steve's business. As his work hours became filled with clients and many other related tasks, Steve found less and less time to do some of the things necessary to grow his business. Steve used the following six steps to figure out who he needed to hire based on what activities he could delegate.

BEING FULFILLED

1) Create a list of all the activities/commitments in your typical business week separated by each day.

2) Determine how appropriate each activity to the success of your business vision.

3) Delete or cut back on any activity you feel unnecessary.

4) With the remaining activities, determine how important it is for you to do each activity on a scale of one to three. One means you must do it; three means someone else can do it.

5) Decide which activities will be hired out to the right people.

6) Find those people and hire them immediately.

Based on these six steps, Steve was able to identify many activities that were just wasting his time, and he was able to delete them from his calendar. He determined that he would hire a bookkeeper to take care of income, expenses, and the financials of his business. He also hired an assistant for ten hours each month to help out with data entry and paperwork. These ten hours were just enough to unload some important tasks so he could use his skills to produce more income. **The largest benefit to having the right people in your business is leveraging some of their energy points to produce more income for you!**

Steve also was aware that in order to create true financial wealth, it was necessary to create multiple streams of income. From reading, coaching, and observing closely people who had done this successfully, Steve realized that human capital was the main ingredient in creating multiple streams of income. This motivated Steve even more to find the right team to support his vision.

Multiple Streams of Income

If you want to swim in the lake of financial wealth, a place where you are completely immersed in fulfillment from your business results, it begins with multiple streams of income. Let's define multiple streams of income as creating profit from multiple sources. Ideally, you create a situation in your business where you work on one "stream" for a bit of time, and, as it grows, you begin to get paid multiple times on that initial effort. Once that initial "stream" is flowing (or cash "flowing"), you can then focus your efforts on another stream, while that previous stream is still producing income.

Example: Steve produced a DVD course from several of his speaking engagements. He worked on it for about two months with the editors and crew to get it out to the marketplace. At the point when the production was complete, Steve began getting paid multiple times on that two-month effort as people purchased it. This one stream of income produced $20,000 a year for Steve. He knew that all he required were five similar streams of income to produce a fairly passive six-figure income!

Let's visually look at multiple streams of income and the importance of creating this in your world. Look at Figure F. In the middle you see "My Bank Account." Let's imagine "My Bank Account" as a lake. What keeps that lake full? Multiple streams of water. In this example, what keeps "My Bank Account" full? Multiple streams of income. What happens if you have *only one stream* of water going into the lake and it is cut off? The lake eventually dries up. If you have only one stream of income, say a job, and you are laid off, your bank account dries up too.

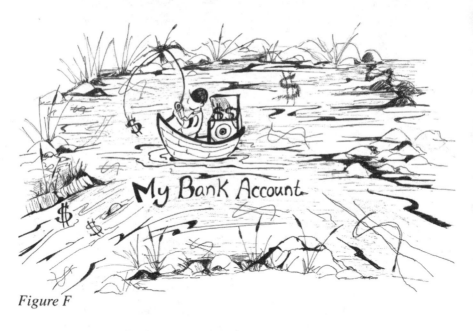

Figure F

3) Hierarchy among Domestiques

Just like Lance Armstrong relied on his "lieutenants" during critical stages, Steve realized that he required people like that in his business as well. These people were the ones that referred heaps of business to him and connected him with big contacts that led to large revenues. Steve's coach always told him that he was one or two people away from a six- or seven-figure income. Steve understood this statement logically, but not experientially because he had not met those people yet. As he continued to grow his database and put people in his pipeline, Steve began to meet some people that he immediately knew were his "lieutenants."

These people not only benefited by Steve's services, but they also sent lots of people his way. They went out of their way to recommend Steve for speaking engagements, and they pulled strings with the connections they had to get Steve in the door. Steve was now experiencing what most entrepreneurs never get to experience: rewards via the big paychecks!

Most entrepreneurs do not stay in the game long enough to experience this. When the going gets tough and they don't see a result quick enough, they drop everything and search for the next best thing. At this point, Steve had stuck to his schedule and new structure for over a year and was just now creating some momentum. He knew he had many more years to go, but the model of investing most of his energy, most of the time in one area was definitely working.

Stage 6:

Maintain Focus on that Vision and from that Vision

Even the most focused people become unfocused. It doesn't matter how it happens, but it happens. **The difference between a successful person and an unsuccessful person is that the successful person takes less time to become focused again.** Because of this fact, it's important that you revisit your vision frequently whenever you require it. Even though you might find yourself consistently moving towards a result, you always are required to see if you are on course.

BEING FULFILLED

It's been said that the space shuttle, when traveling to the moon, is off course 99.99% of the time. In order to get to the moon, the computers are constantly monitoring and making the necessary adjustments. It is your role to ensure that you stay on course because if you are off course 99.99% of the time, it will require too much energy and signals that you do not have a clear enough vision.

Once your vision is strong enough, you will want to keep it in front of you to ensure that you do not take on too many extra, nonrevenue-producing activities. When things seem to be going your way and you suddenly have less to do, do you begin to add useless to-dos and commitments to fill your time?

If you haven't experienced it yet, once your business begins to produce a consistently sizable paycheck, and once your systems are seamless, you might find yourself subconsciously slacking off a little. Even though you are producing results, there might be something deep inside saying, "You made it; you deserve a break." "You can buy this—you are earning more now, and you deserve it." "I don't need to do this anymore; I am past that stage."

STOP! If you slack off now, take a break, or spend more money, it will not be long before you wind up right back where you began: broke, with bad habits, low self-esteem, and no structure. You will then begin to doubt if everything you did was even worth it and want to throw in the towel. Old beliefs will arise and you might even say, "See, I knew it was too good to be true!" At this point, life gets in the way, inspiration seems to fade off, everyone seems to say no, and your days seem to be pointless. You have essentially put your "Poor Me Pity Party" 3-D glasses on. Now everything you look at is popping up pity for you. (The 3-D glasses were outlined earlier under Philosophy #4: Results Are Energy.)

This stage is critical in order that the previous situations do not occur. This is another reason you require a great support network. The right people will keep you focused. If nothing allows you to refocus on your vision, revisit Stage One, and then continue through each stage again to ensure you have done everything possible to streamline your life and focus your energy points appropriately.

Example

For the most part, Steve did a good job remaining focused on his vision and staying true to all he had set up through this process. There were times when he doubted himself, when his old, disempowering beliefs came up. This happened mostly when he compared himself to other people in his industry. He might come across another speaker or coach who just published a book or had mega success at an event. He might see a really cool website and wish his were better.

Steve learned very quickly to maintain focus on his own journey and his own vision. No matter what level he achieved, there was going to be someone bigger and more successful. He began to focus a lot more on this: **Focus on what you have versus what you don't have. Focus on what you have done versus what you have not done.**

Steve reverted back to several of the seven stages when it was necessary. When he found he had trouble focusing, he revisited Stage Four so he could learn about himself better. When he was not producing what he wanted to, he revisited Stage Two where he re-simplified and reprioritized from his vision. When his wife's schedule changed or his business outgrew his organizational system, he ran himself through Stage Three, restructuring and reorganizing his week.

Steve recognized that although these stages were focused around adding structure, consistency, and routine into his world, **the process was also dynamic.** Dynamic does not mean flexible or loose. Dynamic is energetic, vibrant, and active… just like life. Within your structure you will have ups and downs, curveballs and sliders. Being present in the moment and in the flow of life will allow you to release the roller coaster life may bring and keep you producing results with ease.

Stage 7:
Practice and Duplication

"Three times for the normal mind." "Repetition is the secret for success." These were two phrases embedded into my mind in the second grade from a nun named Sister Marie Troy. Any walk of life requires the discipline of practice if fulfillment is desired. Stage Seven is ideally where you want to remain for as long as possible. If you are in this stage, you are consistently producing and staying focused. The moment you are not, go back to Stage Six, refocus, and begin practicing again! There is a simple, three-step formula on practicing effectively:

1) Practice
2) Practice
3) Practice steps one and two again

While you are practicing, you must be keenly aware of how you can duplicate what you are doing and what you have done... especially when you succeed. Most people struggling today have had some success in their lives in the past. Their problem is not that they cannot succeed again, but rather, they cannot duplicate their previous successes. **You must be able to duplicate your success in order to create sustained fulfillment.**

Example

At this stage, Steve was consciously practicing all that he had implemented. Through coaching, he learned that it was important to be consciously aware of each and every action he took each day. For each action, he would ask himself the question: "If I were to practice this action to the point where it became a habit, would it assist or resist my results?" This was a great question to let Steve know if his action was results-oriented or just keeping him busy.

The key to Steve's long-term success was being able to duplicate his successes. To do this, he revisited Philosophy #7: The Fear of Success Is Greater than the Fear of Failure. He knew failure was not the problem—he knew how to duplicate that really well. He began to invest much more time in his successes. After each success, he sat down to figure out what went right and why it happened. He asked himself questions like: "What allowed me to perform so well?" "What strengths did I utilize most effectively for this win?"

He made sure he celebrated before moving on to the next to-do item on his list. Because he invested more time in understanding how to duplicate his victories, his fear of success began to subside. He remembered

BEING FULFILLED

Philosophy #3: Fulfillment Is a Conscious Choice. **He began to recognize the power of creating his own fulfillment on purpose by his conscious decisions.**

What's Next?

At this point, revisit the questions at the beginning of this section and the definition you wrote for business fulfillment. See if you can answer any of the questions differently and more easily this time.

Now that you have read through this section, continue on to the other sections. When finished, if you determine that business will be your main focus, come back to this section and go through all the stages and steps. Know that each stage will take some time to do, and there is no set time frame for them. Be patient and take it one step at a time.

SECTION IV

THE SEVEN STAGES
APPLIED TO RELATIONSHIPS

How to Achieve Unlimited Wealth
via Relationships

Relationship Defined

What is the purpose of a relationship, any relationship? Without meaningful relationships in our life, especially the one with ourselves, *being fulfilled* is not possible. We all want things in life, especially someone to share our experiences with. Many times, especially when you are seeking a mate, you might find yourself in the kind of relationship that you wanted so badly, only to find out it was not what you really wanted. You might find yourself feeling unhappy or complaining.

The problem most of the time is that we don't know what we're after, so when we finally get it, we become disappointed. No matter if you are in a marital relationship, dating, or don't have any relationship to speak of, being clear about what you want from your relationship is essential. In order to become clear you must first understand what a relationship is.

BEING FULFILLED

What is your definition of a relationship?: _____

_____

_____

_____

There is no right or wrong answer. After listening to many answers, a definition that seems to run congruently through them all is: *a relationship magnifies the human experience*. What does it feel like to magnify the human experience? How does it feel experiencing something on your own versus with someone else?

Have you ever attended a large sporting event where the bleachers were packed with thousands of people? When something great happened to the home team, can you remember how the crowd went nuts? There were thousands of people jumping up and down, screaming, with the band playing and lights flashing. People giving high fives to friends and people they did not even know. That is how people magnify the human experience.

On the other end, what if you were the only one in the stadium... what would the energy be like? What if there were only a few hundred people? Have you ever been to a game where the seats were pretty empty? There is a lot less energy, and the experience is not quite the same.

Potential Barriers to Fulfillment

If relationships are so important, why don't people experience what they want on a regular basis? Why are people always breaking up, getting divorced, and losing friends? It boils down to what they are magnifying. People tend to magnify the wrong emotions. They focus on fear, doubt, insecurity, and drama versus love, passion, peace, comfort, and giving. They experience ups and downs, and their relationship becomes a place that has the greatest pleasure and greatest pain.

Do you focus on what is working or on what is not? Unlimited wealth in relationships means discovering a place that you can create unlimited sharing and giving with another person. Things are never perfect, because as Philosophy #6 states: Perfection Does Not Exist. The goal of relationships is to simply strive to create an environment where discussion is open and disagreement is healthy. At the end of the day, realize that you and your partner both have a common goal to lead a fulfilling life with joy and peace and to share that with each other.

What detours people from this fulfilling vision are the rules they create. How about the percentage rule, which says everything must be 50/50 in a relationship? People tend to have unwritten rules that sound like: *"If I do this and you do that, we both can be happy."* But what happens when you feel like you are giving 80% for a long time and the other person is doing less? How long does that last? When your relationship becomes all about who has done what, when it becomes driven by rules and not by love, it begins to die. Everyone needs rules, but in a relationship, you require *roles,* not *rules.*

BEING FULFILLED

Rules and expectations of how things should be done create disappointment, stress, and chaos. How many rules do you have in your relationship? How do these rules magnify the bad moods that follow? Rules direct your focus towards doubt, anger, and who was right or wrong. Through effective communication you can learn to magnify the good emotions by stripping away some of the rules you have learned and created, and you can begin to give without expectations.

When your relationship is a place where you can really give without expecting anything in return, that's when you will receive everything you have ever wanted. Releasing your rules means essentially releasing judgment from yourself and others. This was outlined in Philosophy #5: When You Judge Yourself Less and Trust More, You Will Have Everything You Want.

A loving relationship assists your partner to meet his or her desires and challenges. It means learning to appreciate and acknowledge the other person so you can grow together. One of the main reasons people fall in love is that, in the beginning of the relationship, each person gives the other so much attention... they give the gift of significance and adoration, and they give it freely. When you look in the eyes of an adoring fan, all your needs are instantly met. When someone makes you feel significant, you fall in love, you make a friend, and you build a relationship. If that significance fades, the relationship begins to deteriorate.

Are You Ready for a Fulfilling Relationship?

Once you have determined that your relationship is most appropriately your main focus, invest some time to go through this section. Remember that when you focus on one area, in this case your relationship, most of your energy, most of the time must be here. Please be certain inside your mind that the relationship you wish to focus on is clearly worth your energy and time. Whether you are married or not, you intuitively know the answer to this.

This section can be applied to any relationship you choose. For the purposes of this book, we'll focus on an intimate relationship and on your relationship with yourself. Because of the nature of an intimate relationship, both people must have the desire to make this their focus and go through the seven stages together. When doing this, both of you must decide what will work best to utilize each stage, perform the steps, and answer the questions. If you have a partner who is unwilling to do this with you for whatever reason, don't be discouraged.

This is why going through the seven stages while focusing on your relationship with *yourself* is recommended first anyway. The only way you can love others is to first love yourself. This is called self-esteem, and we will be referencing this throughout the different stages. Once you become clearer with who you are and more comfortable in your own shoes, then you can use this same section to go through the stages with another person special to you.

BEING FULFILLED

Because unlimited wealth means complete fulfillment, it's important to ask yourself some pointed questions so you know exactly how to achieve this in your relationship.

Define relationship fulfillment as specifically as possible:_____

_____

_____

_____

Imagine for a moment that you came across a definition of relationship fulfillment you had written ten years ago. How different would it be from the one you just wrote? How you define fulfillment in this area will drastically change, because throughout your life the people you are with and who *you are* as a person will significantly change. Even though your definition at each stage of your life may look different, see if you notice an underlying, consistent message in each of them. This message will be your true definition that will assist you with keeping the vision you will create in Stage One.

Before we dive into the seven stages, the following questions will assist you in understanding where you are now in the relationship you have chosen to focus on. After that we will apply the Seven Stages to Achieving Unlimited Wealth. The seven stages will assist you in answering all of the questions, so once you go through them, come back and answer these questions.

- *Define relationship success as specifically as possible.*
- *What is your big vision for your relationship?*
- *How clear is that vision?*
- *How well does that vision keep you focused?*
- *How well do you focus?*
- *What is the purpose of your relationship?*
- *Why are you in your current relationship?*
- *Define the results you are looking for in your relationship as specifically as possible.*
- *How happy are you on your own? How does that affect your relationship?*
- *How successful are you when it comes to prioritizing what you want from your relationship?*
- *What specific times have you set aside to be with your loved one?*
- *How flexible is that time? In other words, how often do you allow other activities to replace that time?*
- *What are the main strengths you possess in a relationship?*
- *What areas could you be better at?*
- *What areas do you require yourself to be better at?*
- *How often are you intimate with your partner?*
- *How often would you like to be intimate with them?*
- *If there is a discrepancy between the two, why?*
- *How well have your mastered the art of asking?*
- *How well do you communicate with yourself? With others?*
- *How do you manage stress?*
- *How does stress from any area of your life affect your relationship?*

BEING FULFILLED

- *What happens to your mind (thoughts) and body (physical reactions) when you experience these emotions: frustration, anger, doubt, guilt, feeling overwhelmed, and anxiety? How do these emotions affect your relationship?*
- *How do you deal with relationship success?*
- *How do you deal with relationship failure?*
- *Would you be in a relationship with yourself? Why or why not?*
- *Do you love yourself?*
- *Could you tell someone else that you love yourself?*
- *Define love.*
- *Define what you want from your relationship. Why?*
- *What feelings do you magnify most of the time in your relationship?*
- *If someone were to watch you for a week while in your relationship (or listen to your thoughts), what would they see (hear)?*
- *How would they describe you?*
- *What are some great gold nuggets they would want to duplicate in their own   relationship?*
- *What are some things you do that they would not what to duplicate?*

The Seven Stages to Achieve Unlimited Wealth via Relationships

Stage 1:
Create a Relationship Vision

A relationship is ideally a place where you can be yourself and not have to perform. This state is one of authenticity and truth that only you can define. If you have been pretending for a long time and don't really know who you are or what you want, the answer is not far away. In any relationship, especially your relationship with yourself, truth is found when you break down the walls, let go of the ego, and become honest with yourself—no matter how scary it is.

Relationships are based on trust and on pure, unconditional love which comes when you cease judging yourself. Although judgment must exist in the external world, it does not have to live inside you. We have all used the phrase, "I am my worst critic." Why do you judge yourself so harshly? In order to create a pure vision of the relationship you can have with yourself and others, you must release judgment and accept who you are now.

If you are fat, be fat. If you have zits on your face, own the zits. If you cannot seem to get something right, accept that it is not right. Until you release the judgment that your current situation is "bad" or "wrong," you will remain in resistance with yourself... resistance is pain... and pain is very unfulfilling.

BEING FULFILLED

As you create your vision, the objective is to love yourself so much that you would do anything for you! This vision allows you to put yourself first and give unconditionally to you, like you would to your child. This vision allows you to rely on yourself versus others. When you put too much reliance on other people, they will disappoint you. If you rely on someone else for your happiness, that is a crash course headed for disaster. How can you place your happiness in someone else's hand? **Your fulfillment is your responsibility, not anyone else's.**

Everyone does not have to like you, but you do desire their respect. The same goes for you. You do not have to like yourself, but you must respect yourself. There is a big distinction between the two. While you may not "like" something about yourself… be it the condition of your body or a skill you lack… you absolutely must "respect" yourself. You must respect your choices, your actions, your habits, your morals, and your values.

This self respect is very evident in the "effects" of your life. When you have serious credit card debt, are obese, in an abusive relationship, when you use belligerent language, disrespect others and cross moral lines… all of this is a direct reflection of a lack of self respect. *Any "effect" in your life that is extreme and stands out well below the status quo is a sign of disrespecting yourself.*

How to Create a Clear and Certain Relationship Vision

Any truly fulfilling relationship is built and cultivated over time. This vision is no different. Your success will be derived from working and modeling other people. Just as in business and health we have mentors, coaches, and role models, it's the same for relationships. The best way to create a relationship vision is a three-step process.

1) Find a person/couple who is:
>> *a) Feeling like you want to feel*
>> *b) Expresses the self-respect and unconditional love you desire*

2) Model that person/couple by mentoring, coaching, collaborating, and investing as much of your resources into learning how they do it. This model should provide a vision.

3) Once you to see your vision via their model, create your own model to achieve your vision.

As you invest your time with these people, you will quickly learn the habits and behaviors necessary to feel and express what you desire. Like anything in life, your results will come from learning new habits and discovering an exciting new mindset that will unleash fulfillment forever!

BEING FULFILLED
Example

George is a young entrepreneur who has been married for five years and has twin boys who are three years old. George and his wife make enough money to pay the bills, invest a little and have a few bucks left over at the end of the month for some fun. They own a home and have a short commute to work. George is in okay shape; he considers himself a weekend warrior. He hits the basketball court or the gym two or three times a *month* but is very sore afterwards.

George has looked at his life as a whole and decided that his relationship will be his primary focus. Since the birth of their twins, his relationship with his wife has become very beige. They are great at focusing on the twins, work, and other people... whatever energy is left over, which is minimal, gets tossed into the relationship. They have sex maybe once a month, rarely communicate beyond who is cleaning what or who took out the trash. Both of them have expressed their discontentment, but neither has the time and energy to do anything about it. Every time they have a productive conversation of how "things are going to change," it's never followed through on.

George wants to focus on his relationship because it is distracting him from his business and health. While those two areas are vitally important, George really knows that increased fulfillment in his relationship will allow him more focus in other areas of his life. Even though he would like to get closer to his wife and work with her together on this, he recognizes that he must work on his self-esteem and self-respect first if he truly wants a better relationship with his wife.

George tends to beat himself up. He has never been very confident in any of his relationships. He is uncomfortable with who he is, physically and emotionally. He recognizes that part of developing this self-respect involves working out, eating healthier, and understanding who he is and how he works. George really wants to create a vision, but he honestly has no idea of what he wants or where he wants to go. All he knows is that he just wants to be happier. He used the three steps to begin creating his vision.

1) Find a person/couple who is:
> *a) Feeling like you want to feel*
> *b) Expresses the self-respect and unconditional love you desire*

Because George had no idea of whom or what he was looking for, he simply became more observant of the "effects" in people's lives. If someone was obese or looked like they did not take care of themselves, he knew intuitively knew that was not the person for him to model. Because George was in contact with lots of clients through his business, he was able to ask questions of lots of people. He knew from building a solid business that *the way to connect with people was through asking great questions.*

One day at the office, the phone rang. It turned out to be an old friend, Jerry, whom he had not seen since the twins had been born. Jerry also had two children and had been happily married to his high-school sweetheart for ten years. George could immediately feel his friend's positive and vibrant energy over the phone. Jerry wanted to see how George was and set up a time to get together. George became very excited, because he really missed his friend and he had a feeling that Jerry was going to be his model for creating his relationship vision.

BEING FULFILLED

Over lunch, George became convinced that his friend was the one. Jerry was virtually in the same life situation as George, except he was fulfilled in all areas. Not only did Jerry have a successful business and a healthy mind and body, he was passionately in love with his wife. He spoke about her like it was the first day they fell in love. George had to know how he did it.

2) *Model that person/couple by mentoring, coaching, collaborating, and investing as much of your resources into learning how they do it. This model should provide a clear vision.*

George bluntly told Jerry that he wanted to invest more time together not only to hang out but to learn more of how Jerry achieved this fulfillment. Jerry was more than happy with the idea, so they began investing a lot more time together. George began to see how his friend kept on a tight schedule and maintained his focus. George always knew his friend was focused, but he had no idea how well.

Jerry set aside specific times in his week for his wife, children, family, exercise, and hobbies. At the same time, he kept strict business hours and produced great results. George asked, "How do you do it all?" Jerry replied, "That's just it—I don't do it all. *I focus on the vital few versus the trivial many.*"

George learned that even though his friend loved his family very much, he was not afraid to put himself first. *He took care of his needs and was therefore better able to take care of others.* Receiving was equally as fulfilling as giving. Jerry knew that until his own needs were met, he would be unable to give anything of quality.

3) Once you to see your vision via their model, create your own model to achieve your vision.

George knew where to begin. He was always putting every one else's needs before his and was left feeling empty and angry that no one helped him on the other end. He had the philosophy that "if I scratch your back, you scratch mine." He now recognized that he deserved to scratch his own back first, eliminating all his expectations because he was taken care of. Because of all the "things" that kept George busy in his life, he also realized that if he wanted to take care of himself more, he would have to simplify his life.

Stage 2:
Simplify and Prioritize from that Vision

It might not seem like focusing on a relationship should require most of your focus, most of the time. You may wonder, "Is directing six to eight of my energy points most of the time really necessary?" Think for a moment to a time in your life when you first met the "love of your life." How incredibly fulfilling was that time, and why?

I'm willing to bet you invested every waking moment with that person—either over the phone, in person, texting, emailing, or in your thoughts. Think about when that relationship began to lose its fulfillment (if it has). More than likely, it was when you invested less time and attention in each other. If you want a fulfilling relationship again, you must create it by investing your time.

BEING FULFILLED

A relationship can be a complicated beast, as you may well know. It can be the most fulfilling place, and yet just a minute later, it can be the most painful place. Try breaking relationships down to the five most basic fundamentals and you'll have a difficult time. When you are dealing with the relationship between two unique people, there are so many moments where those fundamentals do not apply and only God knows what to do.

Your relationship with yourself is no different. As you grow and experience different phases of your life, you experience millions of emotions of all different intensities. Even though you might be able to boil emotions down to a basic five or ten, the circumstances and situations can give the illusion that there are a million.

For all these reasons, it is important that you invest most of your energy, most of the time in your relationship if this is your focus. This time is required to fully understand how you and your partner work. Please remember, just like when you have not seen a friend for a long time, if you stop understanding yourself and your relationships for a long time, when you visit them again, it will seem like starting over.

The great news on relationships is that once you attain a certain level of fulfillment, maintaining a steady and unwavering stream of communication, attention, and adoration will sustain this for years to come. This will allow you to put your main focus on either health or business. Assuming your relationship is never neglected, it will remain strong.

In order to begin understanding this process, use the seven steps below. If these steps are focused on your relationship with yourself, there will be more internal than external work. Internal work involves coaching yourself, taking time to journal or meditate... thought-based work. When you go through these steps with another person, you might experience more external work like scheduling more of your time together and communicating.

Seven Steps on How to Simplify & Prioritize from Your Relationship Vision

1) Create a list of all the activities/commitments you do in a typical week, broken down by each day.

2) Determine how many of your ten energy points you estimate each activity takes. Overestimate, because they will use more than you want or think they will!

3) Determine how appropriate each activity is in relation to the success of your relationship vision.

4) Decide which activities must go completely or be cut back on.

5) With the activities you have left, go back to step one and repeat this process two more times!

6) Prioritize your remaining activities/commitments with a ranking of one, two, or three. One is the most results-producing; three is the least. The more you simplify, the more everything will seem like a one. This is how you know you have done a great job simplifying. Add activities that you are not doing but that you know are required, and rank them as well.

7) Communicate necessary changes with appropriate people. Set your boundaries!

Example

If there was one thing George was, it was busy. However, he knew he required focus between work, children, and all the "stuff" he had in his life, because he was always stressed. He began with steps one and two to begin this simplification process.

1) Create a list of all the activities/commitments you do in a typical week, broken down by each day.

2) Determine how many of your ten energy points you estimate each activity takes.

After completing his list, he clearly began to see why he was so overwhelmed. He was more than shocked to see all the to-do items on his list that never got done. On busy days, his total energy points ranged between thirty-five and forty. However, he did have days where he was shocked at how little he really did. Ironically, on those days, he rated his energy points higher and was more exhausted than the "busy" days. George recognized that it was not necessarily physical to dos that drained him; it was all the chatter in his head that pulled him away from fulfillment.

3) Determine how appropriate each activity is in relation to the success of your relationship vision.

4) Decide which activities need to go completely or be cut back on.

George had lots of activities that needed to go. He began with the emotional and abusive chatter in his head. George also weeded out times in his business that were merely fluff and did not produce much revenue. These included some networking meetings, business calls, and

214

internet work. He also delegated much of his busy work to a few of his employees.

He looked at the amount of time he wasted doing errands and making fruitless trips to and from stores. He also noticed that when he and his wife *were* together, they did things like watch television or read, things which really did not do anything for their relationship. He was surprised to find that they had more time together than he imagined; it was just that they did not invest it wisely.

> *5) With the activities you have left, go back to step one and repeat this process two more times!*
> *6) Prioritize remaining activities/commitments with a ranking of one, two, and three. One is the most results-producing, and three is the least.*

Each time George went through this process, it was more revealing. Prioritizing really helped him to see what was most important in his day and how previously those important activities had not been his priority. With this step, George wanted to change the types of activities he did with his wife so they would be more conducive to building a healthier relationship. He also wanted to build in more time for himself.

With the time he cleared from his business and personal day, he was able to add activities for his mental and physical health because he recognized the impact it had on his personal relationship. In addition, he wanted to find a personal coach and schedule more time with his friend Jerry. Jerry also told him of some great seminars, workshops, books, and audio courses that would assist him in developing a more powerful self-esteem.

7) Communicate necessary changes with appropriate people. Set your boundaries!

George quickly communicated and delegated appropriate tasks to his office staff. He talked to Jerry to ask if they could work out consistent times each week where they could meet or talk on the phone. He also talked to his wife to share his ideas about how they could invest their time differently together.

George learned that even though his wife wanted to talk more and have better quality time versus watch television or read, she was just too tired. By the end of the day she was physically and emotionally exhausted from work and the twins. Even though she wanted to give more, she just couldn't—she just wanted to "chill."

This frustrated George a little because he had just learned from Philosophy #3 that fulfillment is not a matter of circumstance, like being tired, but rather a matter of conscious choice. That being said, he rested easy because he knew her focus was first on the children and then her own business which was appropriate. She was already overdrawing from her ten energy points each day, and he knew she required rest. He let go of the frustration by using the energy on himself.

He essentially had to *become the change he wished to see* in the relationship before anything could change. He then communicated to his wife that on several of the nights when they would usually watch television or read, he would be doing other things to help improve his self-esteem. She was fully supportive and a bit relieved. She had expressed feeling guilt that she was too tired to converse, but she just was. Now she was excited that she could rest while George did his thing.

Stage 3:

Structure and Organize Your Days around Your Priorities

You might not think in terms of structure and organization when it comes to relationships, because part of what people love about relationships is that they are spontaneous and unpredictable. While this is very true, once children, business, and everything else in life come into play, realistically, the opportunity to be spontaneous gets squashed down significantly. This does not mean it is impossible, but anyone who has multiple responsibilities knows that structure and organization is essential to relationship fulfillment.

If the thought of having to schedule dates, family time, conversations, and even sex disturbs you... unless you are completely fulfilled, (and your partner is, too) then it's time to challenge that thought. Stage Three is about finding the specific times in your day where you can be with the one you love, whether it is yourself or a significant other. This time, like your business and health time, must be uncompromisable or unlimited wealth will be more difficult to attain.

Six Steps to Structure and Organize Your Day

1) Determine your wake-up time and bedtime each day.

2) Determine your office hours each day.

3) Determine your relationship time and figure out which results-producing activities belong in those hours.

4) Determine your revenue/results producing activities outside your relationship and schedule uncompromisable time for those activities.

5) *Take a close look at your organizational systems in and out of your relationship and begin to improve their effectiveness.*

6) *Stick to your new structure for a minimum of three months.*

Example

George was fully ready to focus on himself. He could clearly see his wife was not in a position to put energy into the relationship, but because he had communicated effectively, he had permission to create his own structure.

1) Determine your wake-up time and bedtime each day

George was pretty consistent with his wake-up time because of the twins. Both he and his wife got up every morning together to get them ready before their nanny arrived. His bedtime, however, was a different story. This was a *big* variable. There were nights he would stay up way too late and regret it in the morning, and there were other times where he went to bed way too early and lay awake for several hours, getting a poor night's sleep. He determined a bedtime of 10:00 p.m. was a good average, and he would see how it worked over time.

2) Determine your office hours each day.

3) Determine your relationship time and figure out which results producing activities belong in those hours.

Because George owned his own business, these hours were a bit flexible. He tended to stick to a traditional nine-to-five day. Because these hours were flexible, George used them as an opportunity to add appropriate results-producing activities in his health and relationship areas.

Once those activities were in place, he then created new office hours, which he cut down from forty to thirty-two. He did this because with more time being invested in himself, he could not work as much without going over his ten energy points each day. George knew this would impact his income; however, he also knew that when he was stronger emotionally, he would be a much better businessman and bring in bigger profits.

4) Determine your revenue/results producing activities outside your relationship and schedule uncompromisable time for those activities.

Because George cut down on his business hours, he was even more aware of the importance of creating uncompromisable time for his revenue-producing activities. Just thinking about these scheduled times allowed him to feel more relaxed. Eventually George discovered that he was able to produce more income in his thirty-two hours than he did in forty because he used much less energy, which produced a greater result.

He set up uncompromisable time for activities like prospecting, following-up, setting up meetings, closing clients, training his employees, and marketing. These were major revenue-producing activities that he could not afford to compromise. Now that he had his business day figured out for the time being, he moved on to his health.

BEING FULFILLED

George was a weekend warrior; he was not very consistent with his health. His simplified schedule allowed some great times to get to the gym and play more basketball. He had always wanted to play in a men's league, but they were at night… usually after the kids were sleeping. As opposed to playing in the league, he would watch television and "think" he was spending time with his wife. Now, because he communicated better with his wife, he was able to add activities, like his basketball league. Just by doing this every week, he felt like a million bucks… after he recovered from the soreness!

> 5) *Take a close look at your organizational systems in and out of your relationship and begin to improve their effectiveness.*
> 6) *Stick to your new structure for a minimum of three months.*

George scheduled his uncompromisable time and worked at it for a few weeks. He thought he had organizational systems in his life, but he was wrong. While he had effective systems in his business, when it came to working out at the gym and his new free time to invest in himself, he would waste minutes at a time wandering around the gym and lose valuable time with his family because the everyday household duties were not getting done. Tightening up his organizational systems allowed him to:

> 1) *Create necessary systems and processes to save time and energy*
> 2) *Establish who does what, when, and how in the house and in the relationship*
> 3) *Systemize his workouts precisely to get in and out with zero wasted time with a killer workout.*

Once George improved the effectiveness of his organization, it was that much easier to stick to this structure for at least three months. He created these systems by working with his coach and talking to other people to see what worked for them.

Stage 4:
Know Yourself and Establish Your New Rules

In a relationship, knowing how you work and what rules you have are important. In the beginning of this section, we mentioned how too many rules in a relationship end up disappointing you and can begin to magnify disempowering emotions. This stage is dedicated to the discovery of those rules and discovering how you tick. The advantage of doing this by yourself is that you can then communicate what you find to your significant other. This will allow them to understand you a bit more clearly so they won't say, "I just don't understand you."

Three Steps to Understand Yourself, Your Rules... and Change!

1) Create an awareness of current behaviors
2) Identify triggers and current rules
3) Consciously practice new responses

Your current habits elicit behaviors that keep you doing the same thing over and over again. Once you identify the triggers and rules that set your old behavior patterns in motion, you can break those old patterns by practicing new responses. In the case of relationships, you don't want to create new rules that will be broken, but rather you want to create guiding principles from your relationship vision. These principles are like a guardian angel that gently reminds you of the purpose you are seeking. Guiding principles cannot be broken like a rule, because they are flexible depending on the situation. Guiding principles recognize that life is not rigid but rather dynamic.

Example

George's schedule was set and he was sticking to it. His vision was clear, time was focused and he was more relaxed. The only thing that seemed to throw him for a loop was his own rules. The more he became aware of them, the more they drove him insane. His rules in and out of his relationship were destroying his energy when he tried to follow them and couldn't.

Example: When one of his children was sick, George could not go to his basketball league. This went against his uncompromisable time. One week he twisted his ankle playing basketball and had to miss his gym time. Because he was so rigid and strict with his structure, when he could not stick to it, like in the examples above, he became frustrated, disappointed, and angry. George was a control freak who was convinced he could change his external environment and the people in it. Through some coaching and reading, he began to let go of some of this control.

Understand Yourself—Emotions

George had a great command over his emotions *when he was in control and everything went according to plan*. Outside of the plan, he was a basket case. He used the three steps and focused them on his emotions.

1) Create an awareness of current behaviors

One behavior that took George out of the game occurred when his family or life did not seem to cooperate with his new plan. He knew that some of it was not his family's fault, like when the kids got sick, but it still caused him to be overwhelmed with fear and anger. Every time he would miss something that was supposed to be "uncompromisable," he would want to give up on everything. He was a bit of a perfectionist—he had the rule of "all or nothing."

If he had an hour to invest with his wife but she could only do fifteen minutes, he would get upset and not do it at all. He found this behavior to be consistent in the areas of business and health, too. If he was late for a workout, he would just bag it all together because it would not be "perfect." If he was bidding on a big job for a customer and they only wanted to do part of it with him, he would throw away the whole deal. He wanted it to be all or nothing.

2) Identify Triggers

George took some time to separate his life into the three categories: business, relationship, and health. With this exercise, he put each category on its own sheet of paper. He then listed all the triggers he could think of that set off his "all or nothing" rule in each of the three categories.

Throughout the next week, he carried those lists with him, and whenever he felt those emotions coming on, he stopped and took the time to write what triggered them.

3) Consciously Practice New Responses

Now that he had a better idea of what his consistent triggers were from the exercise in step two, he was excited to begin practicing new responses. He changed the "all or nothing" rule into a guiding principle: *I will accept and be thankful for what I get.* This instantly allowed him to see some phenomenal results in his life. Before implementing this principle, when George did not get his way, not only would he throw an attitude with others, he would constantly blame and put himself down. This guiding principle allowed George more ease, flexibility, and ultimately more fulfillment, using less energy!

Understand Yourself—Guiding Principles

Guiding principles are designed to assist you to face the challenges of life by developing ideas that support mutual goals and offer long-term, sustainable benefits for everyone involved. Recognizing that people's needs and interests are widely diverse, your guiding principles are developed to be a framework for structuring partnerships and fulfilling relationships versus a set-in-stone set of rules. Three simple phases go into designing your guiding principles:

Foundation

These principles must be built on shared values and philosophies. Whether you are building this with yourself or with another person, these principles should:

1) Begin with an open and frank discussion about values, goals, and needs

2) Respect and reflect the culture and visions of both partners

3) Support the core mission/vision of the couple

4) Bolster the physical, emotional, and spiritual well-being of the couple

5) Clearly define short and long-range visions

6) Focus on collaboration to determine activities that meet the visions of all involved

Implementation

In this phase, you translate the foundation values into action. Communication should be frequent and open to understand each other and yourself on a deeper level. Both parties should be able to "manage" this process and keep each other true to the principles. If necessary, each person should have written descriptions of roles and responsibilities with accountability measures. It's valuable to define specific, measurable outcomes whenever possible to ensure fulfillment.

Evaluation

This phase determines strengths, areas to be improved, and future directions. These evaluations should be done on a regular, agreed-upon basis. Be sure the end result of this evaluation gives specific action and direction to all involved. While this three-phase process might sound mechanical, the formalized steps and written roles will prevent you from assuming something. When people assume and interpret in a relationship, there is little communication and certainty. This leads to miscommunication and failure.

Example

George set up some guiding principles for himself so he could honor his new vision effectively and not be subject to unnecessary rules. He included things like:

- *I value eating well and exercising. I will take every opportunity I can get to choose these activities.*
- *I can trust myself. Only I know what I truly desire, and I deserve to honor those feelings more.*
- *I am only responsible for my own happiness. I will consciously choose to listen to myself more.*
- *Putting myself first is great. I can be intelligently selfish, and I am comfortable receiving.*
- *I will accept and be grateful for what I get.*
- *I will not go to bed angry with myself or my spouse. I will communicate and share how I feel.*

This was a great start for George. The main part to remember is that these principles must be evaluated regularly; they are never black-and-white. Such rigidity can cause unnecessary pain.

Stage 5:
Find the Right Person to Maintain the Focus and Support the Vision

The highest form of relationship outside the one with yourself is an intimate relationship where two people share unconditional trust and truly compliment one another. This partnership, marriage, union, or whatever you choose to label it is the most powerful way to achieve unlimited wealth. For this reason, Stage Five is about finding the right *person* versus people.

In a mutually beneficial marriage, you work as a team for a common vision. You can hire coaches, counselors, and mentors; you can have role models and friends to support you; you can have nannies, maids, chefs, and employees assist you—but nobody can replace that one person who adores you and whom you adore more than life itself. This person will stand and fight for you, and you for them. With this dream team, anything is possible. Two people in a marriage are the vision and dream keepers, while everyone else's energy is leveraged to conserve theirs.

Stage Five as it relates to relationship is not about all the other people you can hire to assist you in your world. This stage is about finding the right person to be on your team. If you are currently in a relationship, married or not, it's important to know deep down that the person you are with is *the one*. How do you know? **You know** by listening to your inner voice.

This is not the voice that expresses irritation or frustration because the other person is lazy or doesn't help out when required. No matter how upset you might be, listen to the voice in your heart that tells you how much you adore and love that person... AND (very important) how much that person adores and loves you. Without recognizing this voice, you are settling for less, and your heart will not be committed 100%.

In a relationship like this, 100% is possible, and it is required. When there is true love, 100% is effortless. You may be angry, frustrated, sad, upset, and disappointed... but at the end of the day your commitment is true and unwavering. Too many people stay in a relationship that is not right because it is easier and less complicated. These are the same reasons why they are in poor health and struggle financially... it is easier and less complicated.

Today the word "commitment" has lost its true meaning. People stay in relationships out of loyalty, not love. If you are in a relationship out of loyalty... if you deep down know that it is not the right one... GET OUT! It does not matter how complicated you *think* it is... the pain of regret that you will carry with you the rest of your life for not listening to your heart will destroy you.

Most people make a commitment and stick with it for a while... and then chicken out. In athletics, you show up every day *no matter how you feel* and put in the time. It takes discipline, hard work, and consistency. The same goes for business, and it's especially true for relationships. You absolutely must be in a relationship that is the right one or unlimited wealth cannot be attained.

Regardless of what kind of team it is, a football team, a business team, or a husband/wife team... if the passion is there, if the communication is there between all segments of the team and all the members are working together towards the objectives, there is almost no way you can fail!

The Husband/Wife Team

With a husband/wife team, *establishing your roles is unequivocally the best activity you can do to consistently move in an intelligent direction towards unlimited wealth*. Who does what, when, where, why, how much, how often, and in what capacity? What are the expectations? How do you communicate? What happens if someone gets sick, tires, is gone, requires assistance, can't do it any more, is feeling overwhelmed? These roles must be communicated frequently. If your focus is business and your spouse's focus is health, how does it fit together? What if it changes? How do you retain your individuality in and out of the team?

Identify, clarify, and communicate. Be open and share. Stop assuming, interpreting, and being silent. Do you revert to childlike behaviors when you're angry? When you are upset and feel the poison inside, do you try and inject that poison purposely into the other person, taking pleasure when they become upset and poisoned? Stop the games and begin to contribute. Pick up the slack if you are the more able one. Stop burying your emotions and sleeping it off. Create guiding principles and honor them. Take the high road, and bring your partner along with you.

Example

George unequivocally knew he chose the right person to be with for the rest of his life. Even though he and his wife could be a lot happier, they both had an eternal light the burned in their souls for one another that could not be extinguished. George realized that his relationship had many unique phases of love that revolved around different responsibilities. One phase of love is not more powerful or weaker than another; they are all equally strong. When he began to accept the phase of love he was in, he was instantly more fulfilled.

Phases of Love

Different phases of love stem from the current responsibilities in a couple's relationship. Below are just a few phases of love that couples can experience. These are here so you can better understand and accept where you are so you are not constantly wishing you were somewhere else.

• **First Love Phase:** This is a place where you first begin to realize you are in love and are being loved back. It is a physical and emotional shift from friend to lover. It is a very distinguishable point in a relationship that only happens once. You can fall in love with the same person over again; however, that is a very different phase because you are so familiar with the person when that happens.

The first love phase is a place where you almost cannot believe the feeling, yet because it is so new and you might not even know that person really well, you just feel so deeply. Typically, this is when all your focus goes into this relationship and other responsibilities take the back burner. In this phase, the other person is indeed perfect and can do nothing wrong.

• **Lusty Love Phase**   Bring it on! This is the phase you often see in the movies. If you are not currently there, you dream of and talk about it all the time. It is where a great weekend consists of not leaving the bedroom, ordering in, and watching three movies where you have no idea what happened in them. This is the most alluring phase once you are beyond it... *and it does pass*. It is alluring because as humans, we have a natural sexual instinct. We are sexual beings, and sex is a primal, fundamental need.

This phase is primarily responsible for breakups and divorce, because when this phase passes in a relationship, it is seemingly very exciting to have again. People will cheat on a spouse to regain this phase. While this phase does pass, it shows up at different times in a long-term relationship, but it typically does not last as long as the first time. Responsibility, reason, and logic are not usually present during this phase, and the other person is God's gift to the earth.

• **Steady Love Phase**   This is the "back to reality" phase. It is like saying, "Okay, I had my fun and really want to continue, but all my friends and family have left me and I am dead broke because I have called in sick every day from work and bought you all the gifts in the world." There is a very strong attraction during this phase. You still cannot get enough of each other, yet it is not as immediate and in the forefront of your relationship as it was in the previous phase. In other words, the first thing you do in this phase might be to go to dinner and then jump into bed, whereas before jumping into bed was obviously the only priority of the day. Here life's normal responsibilities are in effect.

• **The "Roommate" Love Phase**
This phase tends to be prevalent with couples who are raising children, growing careers, and keeping up with everything else in their lives. The majority of those reading this book are most likely in this phase. There is a strong sense of love between the couple, yet there seems to be no time to express it. Intimacy is few and far between, alone time is virtually unheard of, and communication typically is minimal. This is probably the most frustrating time in a relationship, and it's where most couples split. What people don't realize is that this is just a phase, and it's very appropriate give the amount of responsibility they have.

The purpose of understanding the particular "phase" of love you are in is so that the you and your spouse can understand why you feel the way you do and give yourselves permission to recognize that it is normal and okay. Because the model for fulfillment in this book states that you can only focus on one area at a time, how can a couple with multiple responsibilities outside their relationship expect to be in the Lusty Love Phase when they never see each other?

Coming to terms with the phase you and your significant other are experiencing will allow you to grow closer. The challenge here is to sit down with the other person and communicate. Even if the relationship cannot be your main focus at this time, setting up the uncompromisable time outlined earlier in Stage Three will ensure *being fulfilled*.

George also became better at accepting where his wife was in her life. Both of them were working on better communication, and both were excited to establish roles in their world. Because there were so many responsibilities between work, the twins, the house, and many other things, it was refreshing for them to view themselves working as a team. They sat down and went through their day-to-day responsibilities and tasks and divided them all up based on each other's individual and team vision. It was not a 50/50 split but rather what was appropriate. They scheduled a time to meet each month to reevaluate to ensure that both of them were happy. They both agreed to openly communicate their thoughts.

There were times when the roles they established did not work flawlessly, and they easily reverted back to their old ways. Because George understood himself better, there was less conflict and more communication. He learned that communication does not have to be fun or pretty, is just deserves to be done. Stage Five for George was all about ensuring that he was with the right person and taking that to the next level via communication.

Stage 6:
Maintain Focus on that Vision and from that Vision

Life happens, and it can throw even the most focused person upside-down. It does not matter how it happens, but it does happen. Revisit your vision frequently to prevent drifting and becoming busy again. If possible, find a way to keep your vision in front of you with pictures and tangible objects that serve as constant triggers and reminders of what you and your relationship team are going for.

A strong relationship is not born; it's built. It requires constant energy, attention, and focus. Whether your relationship is your main focus or not, neglecting it will allow it to deteriorate… sometimes very quickly. Old habits and behavior patterns, some left over from past relationships, can easily take over again if your vision is not in the forefront of your daily thoughts and activities. A great way to refocus on your vision is:

1) Find outside people who support you

2) Run yourself through some of the previous stages

3) Strategically place tangible triggers to remind you of your focus

The easiest way to maintain your focus is by being true to your thoughts, feelings, and emotions. If you truly listen to yourself and act from what you feel, you will be fulfilled.

Example

Staying with his focus was not easy for George at times. Because his self-esteem was not very high when he began, his inner voice often told him to quit—that nothing he did would work. George used this stage to keep his focus on things that *were* going well versus what was not. He kept reading and learning about personal development. He became a lot more relaxed at home via his guiding principles, and he began to see his wife responding differently. In order to maintain focus on his vision, George learned to celebrate all the small signs of success.

He recognized the smallest little progress with his health, like being one pound lighter or lifting one pound more… and celebrated it. He noticed small signs of affection from his wife and embraced them. He was proud when he had new thoughts in old situations. These new thoughts and perspectives that George was having created a big sense of fulfillment in his life. He realized that his physical world and body did not have to change totally for him to feel fulfilled. All he had to do was adopt a new perspective, release judgment, and be open to new ideas.

Stage 7:
Practice and Duplication

Recognize that you have achieved relationship fulfillment before. Whether you only dated someone for a day or have been married for fifty years, you have felt fulfilled. When it comes time to practice and duplicate in your relationship, go back to the definition at the beginning: *A relationship is meant to magnify the human experience.* Whatever you practice, it must magnify something empowering and fulfilling. You must seek to duplicate the love you experience and desire.

Above all, practice communication. You deserve to understand how you and your partner work as individuals and as a team. At the end of every game, a successful team, whether they win or lose, will sit down and communicate what went well and what could have been better. When a team is on a losing streak, typically it is because they are not focusing on their strengths and big vision. This is when teams get in a funk and begin to expect to lose.

The same goes for your relationships. When you expect to win, you win... even if in reality you may have lost. On a relationship team, each person must understand their own and their partner's strengths. Divide up the responsibilities in your world based on each other's strengths. This will allow you to win more games together and do it using less energy points.

Example

George better understood his strengths and began to practice them, whereas before, all he did was focus on his weaknesses... and on his wife's too. He stopped caring about what he was not good at and began to practice what he was good at. Because he honored this, it was not long before his vision became even clearer in all areas of his life. George also communicated what he learned about himself to his wife. Because of this, she began to accept him for who he was versus wishing he was someone different all the time.

If you are in a relationship long enough, it is easy to wish the other person were better at something or someone different altogether. It is also easier to wish *you* were better or someone different. In either of these situations, accepting yourself for who you are and unconditionally loving yourself will ultimately lead towards unlimited wealth in relationships and beyond.

What's Next?

At this point, revisit the questions at the beginning of this section and the definition you wrote for relationship fulfillment. See if you can answer any of the questions differently and more easily this time.

Now that you have read through this section, continue on to the other sections. When finished, if you determine that relationship will be your main focus, come back to this section and go through all the stages and steps. Know that each stage will take some time to do, and there is no set time frame for them. Be patient and take it one step at a time.

BEING FULFILLED

SECTION V

THE SEVEN STAGES APPLIED TO HEALTH

How to Achieve Unlimited Wealth via Health

The Fitness—Wealth Connection

By this point it is clear that Business, Relationship, and Health all have a direct connection with achieving unlimited wealth. One of these, however, outranks them all in importance of long lasting fulfillment. Unfortunately it's the one that the majority of the population neglects the most: health. Why is health the most important? There is no magical answer besides the obvious one: If you don't have your health, what do you have? It is blatantly simple, honest, and undeniably true. You can resist this until you have a heart attack, and then you will understand the point.

Below are three different life scenarios. Put yourself in each of the three scenarios and pretend it was yours. If you had to circle the scenario you would prefer, which would it be?

BEING FULFILLED

1) A person who is a multimillionaire, terminally ill, who
*   has no friends, family, or significant other to love*
2) A person who is dead broke, terminally ill, who has many
*   close friends and family and is with their soul mate*
3) A person who is dead broke, in perfect health, who has no
*   friends, family, or significant other to love*

Which one did you pick? Can't decide because you want to know more information and details about each scenario? Those are all the details you require. If you want it bluntly, pick one of these:

1) Rich, Dead, Alone
2) Poor, Dead, with People
3) Poor, Alive, Alone

It is fairly obvious that anyone who is not over-thinking this would choose scenario three. The bottom line: *your health is the most important contributor to you being fulfilled.* In scenario three, we eliminated business and relationships and left you with health. Because you have your health, you will have the energy to grow a business and form relationships. **Without your health, you have no hope of attaining unlimited wealth by this book's definition.**

We live in a success-driven world. The majority of those who have not given up or settled on the status quo are working hard at becoming something… at making it big! Take a look at the most popular television programming. Situational comedies have been replaced by reality shows that have a common theme: people competing for an opportunity of a lifetime and large amounts of money. *The Apprentice, Last Comic Standing, American Idol, So You Think You Can Dance, American Inventor,*

America's Next Top Model, Fear Factor, Who Wants to Be a Millionaire?, Deal or No Deal, The Biggest Loser... The list goes on and on.

These shows are so popular because people connect with the contestants. They see part of themselves in that contestant. They see a possible way out of their average lives. The popularity of these shows says a lot about the consciousness of today's society. While people waste precious time watching these shows, it also reflects a society that is more aware than ever before. With books and movies like *The Secret* becoming common house talk, people today are realizing their potential. Because you are more aware of your potential than ever before, it is important to understand what really goes into creating long lasting wealth.

True Health — The Backbone of Wealth

Let's get down to business and talk about your path to unlimited wealth. In order to feel fulfilled in this world, you must begin to stand your ground and speak what you feel. In other words, grow a spine and create a solid backbone for yourself. Take the phrase, *Built to Last*, and apply it to your wealth. As you continue to build wealth in all three areas of your life, what will allow it to endure the ups and downs of your life? Are you building it to last, or just getting it done so you can experience it now?

In our microwave society, the "get rich quick/get fit now" syndrome is based on short term, external solutions. Unlimited wealth is not short-term and external. In order to create wealth with a backbone, we must understand what that backbone is built from. It is built from *true health*. This is not just physical health; it is emotional health as well. True health is based on complete ease within your mind and body. True health understands the basic principles and laws that govern your results.

Jeff's Law of Wealth

When a scientist presents an idea that is not proven, it is called a theory. A theory is not the absolute, entire, and final description. Because it is a scientific theory, it contains certain assumptions and approximations of nature and ultimately fails to describe the theory to a certainty. Great examples are Einstein's theory of relativity and Darwin's theory of evolution. These theories have become popularized as a "scientific truth" because they offer a simplified explanation to the complexity observed in the natural universe, yet they are not the only ways you can look at it. Bottom line, a theory is not proven and is disputable.

Once a theory is proven, it becomes a law. A great example is Sir Isaac Newton's universal law of gravity. This cannot be disputed no matter what you do. Go ahead and jump off a bridge and you will undeniably prove this law. Laws are irreversible and true. *The following is a very important law, which is the foundation of unlimited wealth.*

You *cannot* become healthy by becoming wealthy...
But you *can* become wealthy by becoming healthy.

Health is the wealth sustainer. It may not be where wealth begins; however, it is how it lasts. You can argue that wealth begins with a strong business or a solid relationship... very true. However, when your business or relationship fails for a moment or for good, you must rebuild from your strong physical and emotional health, from your backbone. When your health fails for a moment (or for good), what do you have to rebuild from? Money can buy you the best drugs and doctors. Relationships can give you support and love. They are helpful, yet they provide no backbone for sustained wealth.

242

It is paramount that you understand and embrace the law of wealth just presented. If you resist or work against that, pain is sure to follow. In life, there are rules that we must follow in order to live with ease. Some are common sense and others are less intuitive. Some we have no problems following and others we push the envelope with. It might be easy not to kill anyone, yet you may push the speed limit every now and then. In order to create fulfillment in life, which is the goal of this book, it is imperative you understand and abide by this law.

Unlimited wealth understands that the health of our mind and body has the highest influence over our present energy. Our present energy determines who we connect with and what opportunities we see. Those people we attract and the opportunities we take advantage of will eventually have the greatest influence over our results. Desirable results lead to unlimited wealth.

True Health = Attractive Energy
Attractive Energy = The Right People
The Right People = Desirable Results
Desirable Results = Increased Fulfillment
Increased Fulfillment = **Unlimited Wealth**

It is important to note that true health is not a tight butt or six-pack abdominal muscles… **Just because you look good does not mean you feel good,** but *when you feel good, you look good!* The look is a result of the feel. So, what is true health?

True health is desirable energy created from within which attracts the right people and allows us to see opportunities that will produce a result called complete fulfillment, otherwise know as unlimited wealth.

True Health is Unlimited Wealth.

Your Health Focus

Once you have determined that, in your life right now, health is most appropriately your main focus, invest some time to go through this section. Remember that when you focus on one area, in this case health, most of your energy, most of the time must be here. If you are not sure where your focus is most appropriate—Business, Relationship, or Health—begin with health. If all three are in the gutter, begin here. You absolutely must gain a strong physical and emotional body if you ever want to achieve complete fulfillment in the other two areas.

Now that you know unlimited wealth means complete fulfillment, it's important to ask yourself some pointed questions so you can know exactly how to achieve this in your health.

Define health fulfillment as specifically as possible_____

_____

_____

_____

Take a good look at your definition and revisit it often. As you learn more and grow, your definition will change. Some of my clients wrote that health fulfillment was having a certain body weight or looking a certain way. Most wrote that it was feeling good and having the energy to do things. If you had trouble answering this question, you are not alone. Most people never take the time to define what they are doing, and therefore they lose focus.

The following are some questions you can apply to your health. After these questions we will apply the Seven Stages to Achieving Unlimited Wealth that you have read about applied to Business and Relationships. The seven stages will assist you in answering all of these questions. Once you go through the seven stages, come back and answer these questions.

- *Define health success as specifically as possible.*
- *What is your big vision for your health?*
- *How clear is that vision?*
- *How well does that vision keep you focused?*
- *How well do you focus?*
- *What is your health plan?*
- *How many times a week do you lift weights?*
- *How many times a week do you work your cardiovascular system?*
- *How many times a week to you stretch, do balance work, work your lower back and core muscles?*
- *How many times a day do you create great food choices?*
- *How guilty and out of shape do you feel if you answered "none" to the last few questions?*
- *What are you going to do about that?*
- *How is your overall diet?*
- *Do you diet? If yes, why do you diet, when you know diets don't work long term?*
- *What habits are you creating for exercise and nutrition that will work long term?*

BEING FULFILLED

- *What will your ideal health plan provide for you?*
- *What is the driving motivator that keeps you going every day to stay/become healthy?*
- *How successful is that motivator in achieving the results you desire?*
- *Define your health results as specifically as possible.*
- *How well do you work alone?*
- *How well organized are you? How does this organization or the lack thereof affect your health results?*
- *How effective are you when it comes to prioritizing your health tasks?*
- *Describe the structure of your healthy day.*
- *How successful is the structure of your healthy day?*
- *What are the main strengths you possess regarding your health?*
- *What areas you could be better at?*
- *What are the areas you require yourself to be better at?*
- *How do you manage stress?*
- *How is your mental and emotional health?*
- *How healthy are your thoughts and self-esteem?*
- *What happens to your mind (thoughts) and body (physical reactions) when you experience frustration, anger, doubt, guilt, feeling overwhelmed, and anxiety?*
- *How do you deal with procrastination regarding your health goals?*
- *Why do you procrastinate?*
- *How do you deal with success in health?*
- *How do you deal with failure in health?*
- *If someone were to watch your health habits for a week, what would they see?*

- *How would they describe your days?*
- *What are some great gold nuggets someone would want to duplicate in their health plan?*
- *What are some things you do that they would not what to duplicate?*
- *If you are overweight, why?*
- *What does your extra weight protect yourself from?*
- *Do you expect to be successful long-term in the area of health? Why?*

The Seven Stages to Achieve Unlimited Wealth via Health

Stage 1:
Create a Health Vision

Great health provides you with the ability to fully enjoy life. Great health allows you to do the things you want to do, when you want to do them. Health consists of proper nutrition, exercise, and developing a positive mental attitude via self esteem. To build your health in these areas, ideally you can harness your passions, skills, resources, and preferences into a structure in which you can achieve these.

You are not your health, and your health is not you. Health is simply a condition of your mind and body. Poor health does not mean you are a bad person; it might just mean you have practiced some poor habits and created some poor choices for too long. Revisit Philosophy #2: Great Habits produce Great Results, where we outlined that habits are learned. This means that you simply deserve to create a new habit, not a new you.

The same goes with your health. *Your current health condition is simply an effect of poor habits* and nothing more. "But I am big-boned and have bad genetics." What would happen if you stopped using that as an excuse? Those are circumstances you cannot change. It is to your advantage that you know about them and have even more reason to begin a focused health plan now.

A health vision is more than a goal of losing thirty pounds or fitting into a dress for a wedding. Those are external goals that have no bearing on long-term success. A true health vision will compel you to eat better and work out even when you least want to. This vision is your guardian angel literally dragging you out of bed to hit the gym at five in the morning. Your vision will give you will power and strength even when you are in the worst conditions and circumstances.

You must understand what your health vision is and how it fits into the rest of your life. Just like everything else, health has a place. Most people put health last on their list (if it's even there at all), and this does not work in achieving unlimited wealth. There are appropriate times for doing healthy activities, and we must recognize these times if we desire fulfillment.

How to Create a Clear and Certain Health Vision

Creating your health vision will take time. In the world of health and fitness, the "how tos" of success can overwhelm anyone. One of the easiest and best ways to create a health vision is sticking with this three-step process.

> 1) *Find people who are achieving the results you desire (physical and mental)*
> 2) *Model those people by mentoring, coaching, collaborating, and investing as much of your resources into learning how they do it. This model should provide you with a vision.*
> 3) *Once you to see your vision via their model, create your own model to achieve your vision.*

As you invest your time with these people, you will quickly learn the habits and behaviors necessary to produce what they are producing. In health, it is not specific exercises and foods these people do or eat, but rather the habits and behaviors they possess that you must adopt. In order to grow anything, you must become someone who deserves that result. The more you surround yourself with these people and learn what they have to teach, the more you can begin to formulate your vision and create new habits and behaviors that match that vision.

Be sure to recognize that modeling is not copying. Your model must be your own, not someone else's. **Modeling allows you to see your potential and vision in someone else's model. Once you see your potential, create your own model to achieve your vision.**

A person copying another model exactly is most common with diets. For example, imagine there was a "Dairy Diet" and you knew some people who had much success on it. So you decided to give it a go. Even though you are allergic to dairy, you are determined to model this "successful" diet. So you pound cheese and wash it down with whole milk eight hours a day. Even though your throat is swelling up and you cannot breathe, you tell yourself that you must stick to the diet... This example might sound extreme; however, people do exactly this. The point is, listen to your body and when you look at someone else's model, *create your own from the structure of theirs and make it work for you.*

Example

As we go through these seven stages, we'll use Jenny as an example to show a bit more clearly how each stage is applied. Jenny is the mother of two children, a three-year-old daughter and a six-year-old son. She has been married for several years. She has four siblings, and her dad is still alive. She has neglected her health for many years and is about thirty pounds overweight. Jenny was a competitive athlete in college, and she loved to work out and play different sports. Before the birth of her children, she was a successful entrepreneur. Now that she has become a full-time mom, her husband takes care of the finances and she works about fifteen hours a week with some clients.

Jenny has been at a crossroads for a while. She feels like crap on a daily basis because she is overweight. She wants to be a successful entrepreneur but does not have the time. She also has an average relationship with her husband whom she dearly loves, but she wants so much more. For Jenny, there is not enough time in the day to do everything she is required to and desires to do. Her husband is very focused on his business—he has to be in order to maintain the lifestyle they are used to. She is constantly frustrated and always seems to be in a downward spiral. The one thing that seems to be going well for her is raising her children. Jenny's children are great (for the most part) due to her focused efforts as a parent over the past six years.

Jenny has wanted to improve her health for a long time now. She recognizes her health is the most important aspect and first step in creating her unlimited wealth. After understanding the concepts presented in this book, Jenny recognized that she only has so much energy each day, and that it was being spread way too thin.

With the support of her husband and family, Jenny decided she would become what she termed "a full-time athlete" over the next year. Having been an athlete many years ago, she knows the habits, disciplines, and focus required to be successful in that area. She was excited to use the seven stages to begin her health focus. She began with the three steps to create her vision.

1) Find people who are achieving the results you desire (physical and mental)

Jenny got her big old butt to the health club that she had been donating forty five dollars a month to as an inactive member for the last five years. She had gone there occasionally in the past before a family reunion or a cruise. Because of her occasional visits, she knew a few people and was not a complete stranger to the place. She began taking group fitness classes and using the weight machines.

BEING FULFILLED

Because of her strong entrepreneurial background, Jenny had no problem talking to people. She struck up conversations with the personal trainers, the group fitness instructors, and all the members who appeared to be very healthy. She began to attend seminars and read objective literature on health and how to achieve it. Whenever possible, she connected with the authors and coaches of those writings to see what they had to offer her. She was determined to find the special person who could best assist her.

At one seminar she attended, she really connected with the personal trainer's physical and emotional energy. Jenny immediately knew she found the person who she wanted to model.

> 2) Model those people by mentoring, coaching, collaborating, and investing as much of your resources into learning how they do it.
>
> 3) Once you to see your vision via their model, create your own model to achieve your vision.

They began coaching and training together. Jenny quickly saw a clearer vision of how she could succeed with her long-term health plan. Jenny formed this vision of hers by getting inside the mind of someone with the habits she wanted to adopt. Jenny saw more specifically what she was required to do each and every day if she were to succeed. Even though it was still hard for Jenny to get to the gym and eat better, Jenny knew that once she created this clear and certain vision, it would become easier. The vision would provide the necessary fuel each day to get her doing what she needed to do. At this point, Jenny was clear enough to begin Stage Two.

Stage 2:
Simplify and Prioritize from that Vision

When your health vision is very clear and certain inside, the need for this second stage will become very obvious because you will be motivated to take action, but most likely you will not be able to fit that action into your hectic life. The objective here is to simplify your day down to the results-producing activities necessary for your fulfillment. This simplification process is designed to rid your time of activities that merely keep you busy and direct it towards results-producing activities that keep you focused. Remember Philosophy#9: Become Focused, Not Busy.

When it comes to health, the one key component that is most often overlooked is your emotional health. The physical components that do not serve you will be easier to spot. It is your main duty at this stage to identify the emotional commitments you have that unnecessarily usurp these points. This is why it is so important for you to embrace the fact that you only have ten energy points each day. If most of your points, most of the times are to be invested in your health; emotional commitments that distract you from this focus **must be deleted** from your day.

Once you have identified the areas that need to go and the ones that deserve to stay, prioritizing these activities is a must. You may not know what all these activities are yet, and this is why it is important to work closely with a coach or mentor who can assist you in discovering what works for you.

Seven Steps on How to Simplify and Prioritize from Your Health Vision

1) *Create a list of all the activities/commitments you do in a typical week, broken down by each day.*

2) *Determine how many of your ten energy points you estimate each activity takes. Overestimate, because they will use more than you want or think they will!*

3) *Determine how appropriate each activity is in relation to the success of your health vision.*

4) *Decide which activities need to go completely or be cut back.*

5) *With the activities you have left, go back to step one and repeat this process two more times!*

6) *Prioritize remaining activities/commitments with a ranking of one, two, and three. One is the most results-producing, and three is the least. The more you simplify, the more everything will seem like a one. This is how you know you have done a great job of simplifying. Add activities that you are not doing but that you know are required, and rank these as well.*

7) *Communicate necessary changes with appropriate people. Set your boundaries!*

Example

Jenny was very overwhelmed with all she had to do each day. Even though she began working out and eating better, trying to fit more into her already busy day was not working. She had dieted and exercised in the past and had experienced the yo-yo effect many times. She was not about to do that again, and she knew she was spreading herself too thin. For Jenny, it was not the physical commitments that drained her; it was the emotional ones. Stage Two was very necessary. She ran herself through the seven steps to simplify and prioritize from her vision, and came up with the following:

> 1) *She created a list of all the activities/commitments she did each day in a typical week.*
> 2) *She estimated how many of her ten energy points each one took.*

At first, Jenny resisted creating this list. She thought she knew all her commitments and had a handle on her activities. She just wanted to begin scheduling. Even though Jenny was overwhelmed with all she had to do, she prided herself in "doing it all." In some ways, she felt like she "had to" do it all. Despite her resistance to step one and two, Jenny did them and surprisingly discovered how much energy many of her commitments actually utilized.

For instance, Jenny loved being involved at her children's school, and she helped out with a lot of activities. She also volunteered to drive other children to and from sporting events and daycare situations. In addition, she squeezed in about fifteen hours a week with her clients because she loved to earn money and loved being and entrepreneur. After seeing all this on paper, the stress of all these activities was overwhelming.

Creating a list of every activity you perform each day with an energy rating next to each one is very similar to keeping a food log. Many people going on a serious nutrition or training program keep a food log of everything they eat over a certain period of time (three days or more). Next to each food item, they put how many calories that item contained and when it was eaten. With an accurate food log, not only can you see the total calories you have consumed, but you can also identify patterns in eating, the time frames, the types of foods, and the quality of nutrients each possesses.

While a food log can be tedious and boring, it will almost always produce a huge surprise and a valuable lesson for the average person. Most people have no idea how many calories they consume each day. When asked to guess, most underestimate by at least 400 calories or more. Four hundred calories is only one piece of pizza! Underestimating and overeating by only 400 calories each day can result in gaining over forty pounds in a year! Investing your time in an accurate physical and emotional activities and commitment log can create all the difference in the world.

It was now even clearer that if Jenny wanted to succeed, she would have to drop many of these activities from her week, but which ones? Even though she genuinely loved them all, her total energy point ratings averaged over fifty each week, which is a lot more than ten... and she felt the effects of that too. She proceeded to the next few steps.

3) Determine how appropriate each activity is in relation to the success of your health vision.

4) Decide which activities need to go completely or be cut back.

5) With the activities you have left, go back to step one and repeat this process two more times!

Even though cutting back on activities was difficult for Jenny, her vision was her saving grace because through it, she saw a way out. Creating her activities list and investing in sessions with her life coach, she identified that many of her activities just kept her busy and distracted from her true health goals. Doing this also protected her from failing at her health goals again.

Because she had yo-yoed with her weight and emotions so many times in the past, there was something inside her that did not expect she could actually succeed. Instead of facing that fear head-on, she buried it and protected herself by committing to everything under the sun. This was all subconscious until coaching brought it out. She now realized that her commitments gave her a valid excuse why she could not succeed. She really did not have the time and energy to lead a healthy lifestyle.

By weeding out all these busy time commitments, she would now have no excuse as to why she could not succeed at her health goals, and she would have to face her fear head-on. She knew that succeeding would build her self-esteem because she relied on herself. In the past, she relied on other people and diets for her success and esteem. Inevitably, they all let her down.

Jenny began to drop the majority of her driving and volunteer work. She eliminated phone calls she regularly made, dinner parties where she overate, and she even decided to step down from her position on the parent-teacher association. She looked at her fifteen hours a week as an entrepreneur and cut back on some clients. Cutting down on these commitments released a huge weight inside Jenny. She could already see her vision being achieved with more certainty.

The best part in eliminating these activities was that Jenny could see a way out of this downward spiral. She finally saw a way to achieve the things she *really* wanted in life… like a more fulfilled marriage, quality time with her kids, and most importantly, a healthy relationship with herself!

Jenny continued through the first four steps a few more times and cut down on even more activities, like the time she spent with friends and outside family members. She also removed the unnecessary things she did around the house. Jenny was a bit of a "perfectionist" and tended to waste time trying to improve something that was already fine. Practicing Philosophy #6: Perfection Does Not Exist allowed her to cut unnecessary activities more easily.

6) *Prioritize remaining activities/commitments with a ranking of one, two, and three. Add activities you know you need to do but are not doing.*

7) *Communicate necessary changes with appropriate people. Set your boundaries!*

Jenny had a fire inside that made these next two steps easier. Note: *It is one thing to cross activities off your list, and another thing to communicate to others what you are doing.* She created a list of all the people she planned to call and speak to about deleting activities. When she spoke to these people, she was clear and did not beat around the bush. She stated how she was not going to do "x" activity as of next week, and she appreciated the opportunity to let them know.

It was amazing how people understood! She thought they would give her a hard time, but they did not. Most people admired her for what she was doing and wished they could do the same. Jenny replied with a smart, "Stop wishing and begin doing!" With all this newly created time, she added in the necessary workouts and activities that would ensure her fulfillment with her health vision.

Stage 3:
*Structure and Organize Your Days
around Your Priorities*

When it comes to health, unless you are a professional athlete like Lance Armstrong whose whole day literally focuses on training (get up, eat, train on bike for six hours, eat, stretch, athletic massage, review ride stats/performance, plan for next day's training), then you might not require more than two to four hours *each day, five to seven days a week* to achieve your health goals. If two to four hours *seem like a lot*, you are underestimating what a health focus truly takes to be successful.

With two to four hours required each day, some of your day will be open for other activities. This is where you must choose wisely. Great physical and mental health requires recovery time and great nutrition that fuels the changes. You can be on the best training program in the gym, but if you don't have the proper recovery and nutrition, your success is very limited.

Six Steps to Structure and Organize Your Day

1) Determine your wake-up time and bedtime each day, which is even more crucial for proper recovery.

2) Determine your "health" hours each day.

3) Determine your results producing activities (workouts, meals) and where they should occur during your day.

4) Determine your results/revenue-producing activities outside your health focus and schedule uncompromisable time for those activities.

5) Take a close look at your organizational systems in and out of your health focus and begin to improve their effectiveness.

6) Stick to your new structure for a minimum of three months.

Example

After all her energy-zapping commitments were deleted, Jenny sat down and created a structure geared to her health fulfillment. She used what she had learned from seminars, books, and her personal trainer to create an effective structure for her weeks using the six steps.

1) Determine your wake-up time and bedtime each day, which is even more crucial for proper recovery.

Jenny previously was getting up at 4:30 a.m. and usually did not hit the sack until 10:00 or 11:00 p.m. each night. She got up so early and went to sleep so late because it was the only time she could find to try and keep up with all of her to-dos. She recognized that those hours drained her and went against her health goals. She decided to get up at 6:00 a.m., which felt like sleeping till noon for her, and go to sleep by 9:30 p.m. With the type of workouts she was going to be doing, her body craved the rest.

2) Determine your "health" hours each day. How long do you have for health?

Since the finances were her husband's focus and he supported her on this, she did not "have to" work. There was a huge part of her that wanted to, but she recognized there would be a more appropriate place for that in the future. Her main focus was her health, and after that she put her remaining energy into her children and supporting her husband with his focus. Jenny structured between three to five hours each day, taking Saturdays completely off, for her health time. This was specific time where she would *only focus* on her physical and emotional health.

BEING FULFILLED

3) Determine your results producing activities (workouts, meals, meditation, etc.) and where they should occur during your day.

Jenny incorporated strength training, cardiovascular work, and group fitness classes at her health club. She also structured in yoga, Pilates, massages, reading, meditation, and outdoor activities. She scheduled more pedicures and shopping time with her girlfriends, relaxing activities that she really enjoyed! She looked at her schedule and, with the help of her coach, implemented these into her week fairly effortlessly. While doing this, she came across some conflicts and activities she had not deleted or cut back on yet. She simply revisited the previous stage's steps to simplifying and was on her way.

4) Determine your results/revenue producing activities outside your health and schedule uncompromisable time for those activities.

Uncompromisable Business Time

This was an area that Jenny cut back quite a bit on. Even though she really wanted to grow her business and wanted it to become a major focus some day, she knew that now was not the *appropriate* time. She cut back from fifteen hours each week to only six. She scheduled a three-hour block on the two days where she did not have as much family or health time planned. She began the process of releasing the "need" to grow her business *now* and placed her focus instead on the fact that she was still taking appropriate steps, just much smaller ones. This helped unload lots of stress and cut way down on valuable energy points being wasted each day.

Uncompromisable Relationship Time

Jenny's time with her children was chaotic and lacking quality. Jenny found that by getting rid of the volunteer and driving activities, she was able to find precious time alone with them more often. By not having four kids in her van, Jenny was able to actually talk to her own children. Also, by having someone else drive her children home, Jenny was able to finish other duties so when her children arrived she was not multitasking, but rather able to be with her children. This was very different and very fulfilling.

When Jenny boiled it all down, she was actually spending about three hours *less* each day with her children… however she felt 100% more fulfilled! She could see clearly that her children felt the same because they began to listen more, and her son actually told her he was happier. That warmed her heart! Perfect reinforcement for the phrase *quality not quantity.*

Jenny and her husband also were growing closer. Because he supported her focus and she supported his, they felt more like a team versus competitors. They structured family time, which consisted of eating dinner together and going for walks with the children. Jenny and her husband also scheduled one time each week when they met for lunch and had a little date. This was something they both looked forward to and never compromised. Their commitment to each other increased, and so did their love and fulfillment.

The key to Jenny's fulfillment was that these times were *uncompromisable.* She was a very disciplined woman who knew the value of sticking to a schedule already from being a great mom. She had seen how well her children worked from sticking to a schedule, and she wondered why it took her so long to realize that she would benefit from a schedule, too! Jenny could already sense that she was producing more from each of her ten energy points.

> 5) *Take a close look at your organizational systems in and out of your health focus and begin to improve their effectiveness.*

While executing her new structure, Jenny noticed many organizational things that slowed her down. Her home and car were a complete mess. Her children's rooms were even worse. Getting the children ready for their day was so time-consuming because she could not find what she wanted. The mess that she lived in was constant feedback of how chaotic her life had become. More than physically slowing Jenny down, these messes drained her emotionally as well.

Even when she began to feel more fulfilled, she would get into her car and sigh from the mess. She would walk into her house and feel overwhelmed and disgusted. Step five allowed her to get the whole family together to organize and clean their external environment… and begin to keep it that way.

> 6) *Stick to your new structure for a minimum of three months.*

Even though Jenny's vision motivated her, she had not created new habits yet. She knew from the ten philosophies outlined earlier that motivation was like a sugar high. Her success would rest upon the new habits she was creating. Philosophy #2: Great Habits Produce Great Results was key. The power of repetition and knowing that what we focus on grows allowed Jenny to keep her uncompromisable time and stay on schedule.

The three-month time frame recommended in step six is crucial, because this is the time frame where new habits begin to stick. No matter how great you feel, slacking off or going back to an old way even for a day can very quickly rekindle an old habit practiced for thirty years. We have all heard of someone who quit smoking for a long time and then decided to "just have one" and suddenly was smoking all the time. Old habits die hard; if you are serious about fulfillment, long-term must become a part of your vocabulary.

Stage 4:
Know Yourself and Establish Your New Rules

Now that you have simplified and prioritized from your vision and have created a structure around it, it's necessary to understand how you perform in this new environment. How do you operate under different situations? An example: It's five in the morning, and your new structure says get up and hit the treadmill in your basement. You are tired, cold, and the bed is very inviting. What do you do?

How do you react when you have been "sticking" to your structure for a while, yet haven't seen any results? The odds for fulfillment are not in your favor. If you don't know how you operate, pray the airbags go off once you hit the wall.

Leveraging Your Resources and Values for Health

A client, Patrick, wanted to begin his healthy lifestyle. Patrick was a very successful entrepreneur creating great profits from his enterprise; however, it had cost him his health and relationships to do so. He had fifty pounds to release, lower back and knee problems, high blood pressure, and high cholesterol. In addition to all that, he had some really bad habits. His diet, while very tasty, was not even close to healthy. He did not exercise, and even when he tried, he was limited to what he could do because of his injuries.

He did not mess around when he did something. Patrick joined a health club, hired a personal trainer, a personal chef, and a personal coach. Even though Patrick recognized the great need for change and had a killer team around him, something still was not working. He would blow off the personal training appointments so he could work. Even though he would forfeit the money, he knew he would make more money by working.

He would forget to take the meals to work prepared by the chef, causing him to rely on his poor eating choices each day. He was also in the habit of getting fast food on his way home from the office. Because of this, he would get home to a nicely prepared, healthy meal, and not even be hungry... but he ate the meal anyway!

What was missing was a way to *ensure* Patrick's success. We had to find a way to leverage his resources and values to overcome his current habits. If there was one resource Patrick had, it was a lot of money. Even though he had lots of it, he was very tight with it and hated to spend it, so we used this to his advantage. Here is how we leveraged his resources and values with his personal trainer.

For every ten sessions, Patrick handed over five thousand dollars in cash to his personal trainer, *in addition* to the cost of the ten sessions. Each session that Patrick attended, the trainer would give Patrick five hundred dollars back as a "reward/payment" for working out. Each session that Patrick missed, the trainer would keep the five hundred for himself! Why? Patrick figured his time to be worth three hundred dollars an hour. Before, he would easily miss a personal training session for work because he could rationalize it with money. He instantly lost that rationale with this setup.

Patrick valued earning money, and it was an important resource for him. By creating a situation that leveraged these values and resources, he did not have to fight his old habits and as a result, simply showed up to his sessions without struggling or thinking about it! The first part of success is showing up every day. If you are finding that to be the most difficult part, leverage your resources and values like Patrick did.

BEING FULFILLED

Three Steps to Understanding Yourself, Your Rules... and Change!

1) Create an awareness of current behaviors
2) Identify triggers and current rules
3) Consciously practice new responses

Create an awareness of what is keeping you doing the same thing over and over again. Identify the triggers and rules that set your old behavior patterns in motion. Then break those old patterns by practicing new responses and creating a new rule book. Create rules that serve you versus those that hold you back. Challenge everything you know to see how it fits into your new focus.

Example

Jenny was well on her way to new habits and greater fulfillment. The only hiccups she noticed were how she felt when she was knocked off her new routine. When things went as planned she was fine, but when someone or something (like "life") did not cooperate, she would be sidetracked.

Jenny definitely required the most work to understand her emotions, especially those around eating. She realized she was an "emotional eater," but really had no idea what that meant. Understanding herself and what triggered her to "emotionally eat" was the key to success.

For Jenny, food had become a substitute for love and fulfillment. Even though she had felt more fulfillment lately with her new structure, she was not even close to the results she desired. She thought that what was lacking emotionally could be instantly filled physically with food. Before she realized what had happened, she had created a cycle of binge eating that ironically left her feeling both physically and emotionally unfulfilled.

ContrAddiction

People become addicted to many things in life. Let's go beyond the obvious like alcohol, nicotine, or marijuana. What about sex, working, eating, or spending money? Let's go even deeper than that and recognize that what people are really addicted to are emotions. An addiction means that you are using an activity to avoid or fill another area in your life you are uncomfortable with or unfulfilled in. You rely too much and too frequently on that activity to substitute and replace the real thing. This happens mostly because obtaining the real thing seems too hard, scary, or painful to create from your perspective. As a result, you find something you are good at or really like and dive into it even more.

People don't get addicted to the action per se, but rather the chemical release that action releases in our body. This is what I mean when I say people are addicted to emotions. Emotions are simply the result of a chemical release. Let's look at how this works with a chemical in our body called adrenaline.

When you hear a motivating song, get spooked walking down a dark street, or even suck down your ten-dollar Starbucks, adrenaline is released, and you feel a surge of energy as your heart rate increases and you became more alert. In our bodies, every encounter we experience produces a feeling. *That feeling is a result of a chemical reaction.* When we practice an action frequently enough, we not only get good at the specific action, but we become "addicted" to the chemical released as well.

People that drink coffee each morning are not addicted to the coffee or even the caffeine. They are addicted to the chemical released from the *thought* they have when they think about drinking coffee and are actually drinking the coffee. They become addicted to the chemicals released when they think about how coffee will temporarily release them from their stressful morning or wake them up. That is why simply *the thought of not having a coffee* each morning will throw someone out of whack. They don't require the caffeine, they require the drag from the chemical the thoughts of having the caffeine produce.

Watch an avid coffee drinker simply thinking about their morning coffee. Listen to them talk about what it does and see how refreshed they look before they even have the coffee! Before they even drink it, they are taking hits off the chemical released from thinking about it! The actual drinking is merely carrying out a clear and certain vision they had in their head.

The interesting part about most additions is that they typically contradict what a person wants in his or her life. For example, a person might work out so hard, wanting to get healthy, yet use unhealthy food to replace a defeated feeling of failure. This is what I call Contr**Addiction.** The addiction contradicts the very result the person desires.

This is why it is important to allot no more than six to eight energy points each day to your main focus. If you find you are consistently at a ten in one area, it's a sign of one of two things:

*1) You are simply neglecting the other two
    areas unknowingly and are heading for
    greater pain via regret down the road.*
*2) You are avoiding something you perceive
    to be painful in one or both of the other
    areas.*

Now that you are more educated about what you might be doing, take an honest look at why you might be addicted to something. Begin to create the appropriate changes using the seven stages and the ten philosophies outlined earlier.

BEING FULFILLED

Jenny used the three steps to create new behaviors.

1) Create an awareness of current behaviors

After every workout at the health club when she finished showering, Jenny would step on the scale. She saw some results, but most days they did not happen quickly enough. On the drive home she would go into her head, thinking about how this was not working and thinking that she was probably better off just quitting. She would immediately try and shift her thoughts to feel better and think about what she would do when she got home. All she could see was herself digging into a bag of chips hidden in the closet.

Before she knew it, she was holding the empty bag of potato chips in the air shaking the remaining crumbs into her mouth. She had polished off the whole bag to stuff those defeated emotions she had in the car, and now the real emotions would fly. The guilt, anger, and depression kicked in because she was working so hard, investing so much time and money into her health, yet sabotaging it all with her eating. All this pain was a result of attempting to replace a sad emotion of not seeing a good enough result with poor food choices. These mood swings released chemicals like cortisol, which kept her overweight despite all her hard work.

2) Identify triggers

Jenny discovered two triggers that caused her to overeat. The scale was one. The second was when her husband arrived home from a business trip. She would be all excited to see him, but he would walk in the door exhausted and complaining. She became disillusioned about him being thrilled to see her and wanting to talk. She stuffed that disappointment with food.

3) Consciously practice new responses

Jenny began to stay away from the scale. This was not easy at first until she began to experience the benefits from it. She set herself up for success after she showered at the gym by walking a different way back to her locker so she would not even see the scale. She also told someone in the locker room that if they saw her go near the scale, they were to say, "Don't you dare!" Now when she was driving home, she was better able to focus on how great the workout was and how good she felt. When she arrived home, she ate much better and did not crave the chips, even when her son ate them in front of her.

She also communicated with her husband about the trigger he unknowingly caused. They came to an agreement that if he was feeling tired and down, he would call before he got home to give her what they termed a "mood barometer." Even if he was in a bad mood, they could now joke about it, and as a result, her binge eating disappeared.

Jenny created new rules from these new practices:

I don't have to weigh myself to know I am feeling and looking better.

I don't have to be with my husband immediately when he comes home from a trip.

Just because my husband is tired and in a bad mood does not mean that he is not thrilled to see me.

She also realized that she did not "have to" buy chips and cookies "for the kids." She learned that the kids only ate them because they were there; they did not require them. Once Jenny stopped buying them, after a few weeks her kids did not even miss them... and neither did Jenny!

Stage 5:

Find the Right People to Maintain the Focus and Support the Vision

When it comes to your health focus, having the right people around you is essential even if you think you know what to do. If top athletes like Lance Armstrong require a team around them even though they know what to do… you do, too! Here is where it can be easier to use circumstances to bail you out like, "I don't have the money" or "I don't know the right people." If you find yourself doing this, direct yourself back to Philosophy #3: Fulfillment Is Not a Matter of Circumstance; It Is Largely a Matter of Conscious Choice.

Not only will you require the right people inside your health focus, like personal trainers, nutritionists, and personal coaches, but you will also require people to assist you with the rest of your life as well.

Example

Jenny was well structured and simplified her life quite well. In order to really execute this simplification process and clear her schedule, she required the right people to step it up and assist her. Stage Six was paramount for Jenny to maintain what she had already created and to take her results to the next level. Jenny used the concept of the domestique outlined in the business section to implement the right people into her world.

1) Basic support

There are six steps you can utilize in finding the right people *outside* your health focus:

1) *Create a list of all the activities/commitments you do each day in your typical week that pull you away from your health focus.*
2) *Determine how appropriate each activity is in relation to the success of your overall fulfillment in life.*
3) *Delete or cut out any activity you feel is unnecessary.*
4) *With the remaining activities, determine how important it is for you to do tha activity on a scale of one to three. One means you must do it; three means someone else can do it.*
5) *Decide which activities will be hired out or delegated to the right people.*
6) *Find those people, hire them, and enlist them immediately.*

The largest benefit to having the right people outside your health focus is using their energy points to do your outside tasks so you can direct most of your energy to produce bigger health results for you.

With two children, Jenny had major responsibilities that she had been doing herself for over six years. Not only that, she was responsible for other people's children as a driver, getting them to and from activities. In addition to that, with all the volunteer work she was doing by being a leader in the community, people relied on her.

She used this to her advantage and turned the tables. Because people had relied on her so much, it was her time to rely on them. She began to ask for what she wanted, and people bean to respond. This *receiving* was very different from Jenny *giving* all her time and energy. Jenny began understanding the value of keeping her precious energy versus carelessly giving it out to anyone.

Zig Ziglar said, "If you help enough people get what they want, you can have everything you want." Jenny had helped enough people get what they wanted and now she was ready to reap the reward. So what did she do? She asked the parents of the children she had assisted for so long to take over the driving responsibilities. She asked some of her local siblings and her dad to assist her. She used the power she had as a leader in the community to essentially show people their new roles as she took herself out of the picture. She became great at focusing on herself. **Most people will not succeed in business, relationships, and health, because they are so good at doing things for other people but not for themselves.**

2) Tactical support

Once her responsibilities were taken care of outside her health focus, tactical support took place *inside* her health-focused world. As she began to see better health results, she knew she required herself to work smarter and effectively. Anyone can start an exercise program and feel better. When you get closer to your bigger vision, however, it requires a bigger mindset and better people. This is where she enlisted the services of a personal trainer.

Though she could not afford to use him each time she worked out, she found a way that he could keep her accountable to get the workouts done, and she used his expertise to program her workout. In some of the group fitness classes she attended, she got to know the instructors and participants well enough so that when she required advice and support, she could easily ask for their time.

3) Hierarchy among domestiques

Just like Lance Armstrong relied on his "lieutenants" during critical stages, Jenny realized that she required people like that in her health focus as well. These people were the ones who she could trust the most. These people were ones that could be completely objective and honest with her when she needed it, but also supporting and nurturing when necessary. Jenny found a life coach that provided all of this and so much more for her. Her coach assisted her with her thoughts, with understanding some of the triggers previously discussed, and with empowering her to implement the change she wanted to see. The objective and nonjudgmental environment they created together was a sanctuary she could not find anywhere else.

Jenny also found a woman at the gym who had similar goals and visions. They became great friends and empowered each other to rise to the next level. It was truly a mutually beneficial relationship where both equally supported each other and allowed each other to grow. Jenny also found valuable opportunities to communicate with her husband as he was going through a similar process with his business. Their relationship became stronger as a result of this open communication.

If you take five of your closest friends and averaged their yearly income, that is about how much you earn in a year. If you compare the quality of your relationship with your five closest friend's relationships, odds are, they are similar. If you take five of your closest friends and average their weight and health status, that is about what you weigh and how you feel. Bottom line: **You become like those you hang around with the most.**

This is especially true in the world of health. No matter what the condition of your current health is, what would happen if you lived in a house for five years with people that were a hundred pounds overweight? What about living in a house for five years with professional tri-athletes? The answer should be obvious. If you are looking to become healthier, you must begin to invest most of your time with people that are in better shape than you are. Being the slowest one of the bunch might not feel great; however, it will absolutely get you serious results.

Stage 6:
Maintain Focus on that Vision and from that Vision

When you lose your focus, how long does it take you to refocus? This stage ensures that you maintain focus as much as possible. When it comes to physical and emotional health, it is easy to lose focus, because there is so much information out there that can confuse you. In addition to information overload, if you experience an injury, which most active people will at some point, being able to create ways to maintain your focus is essential.

Once results begin to happen, it will feel tempting to add activities back into your schedule that you previously took out. Once you drop some weight, it's easy to add poor food choices as celebrations or rewards for a job well done. Any time you do this, however, you are moving away from your focus. Six months may feel like a long time, but it is not. Two years may feel like forever, but it is not. You goal is to maintain your specific focus and maintain it with as little effort as possible for as long as you can. In the area of health, as long as you can means for the rest of your life!

This stage will also determine if you have truly found the right people. The right people will assist you with maintaining your focus. Be clear about what you expect from each person… when and how they can assist you. Also, be aware that even though you have friends and family that you feel "should" be supportive, they may not be.

Watch Out for the Dream Slayers

Have you ever felt like you were achieving great results in a certain area of your life when someone came along and gutted that feeling instantly? Example: A fifty-year-old client of mine had been working diligently on her health for over three years and had not only released forty-five pounds, she had improved her self-esteem and confidence a hundredfold. She was now looking and feeling better than she did in her twenties!

One day, she came across an old friend whom she had not seen in a while. The first thing her "old friend" said was, "Boy, you look emaciated! What have you been doing to yourself?" That comment ended the conversation.

These people are called "Dream Slayers." They are either really stupid and think the word "tact" is something you use to pin a poster up with, or they genuinely hate to see people feel good and they gain pleasure in slaying that feeling. The worst part is that these dream slayers are very often your closest friends and family. This is why all these stages are critical to your fulfillment. You must understand who the "right people" are. You deserve to understand how you work from Stage Four. If you are easily "gutted" by even the most innocent comment, you must be more selective with whom you share you vision and successes with.

Example

Even with the great job Jenny did with her support structure, she quickly found out she did not have all the right people. She was someone who required positive feedback all the time, and some people very close to her did not provide what she thought they would. Jenny learned *a fundamental rule that is true of all humans:* **When an expectation is not met, disappointment soon follows.** When Jenny relied too much on other people and expected their support, she was disappointed when this expectation was not met. Through her pain, Jenny learned to communicate better what she expected and whom she expected it from.

Because she understood herself better day by day and she honored the fact that the seven stages were a dynamic process, she was able to maintain her focus. She discovered a new trigger every day, learned new philosophies, and created new rules. *She became a student of her own success.* She recognized that everyone she came across was both her teacher and her student. All of these experiences were paramount in keeping her focus on her health.

This stage was particularly important because results with our minds and bodies take time. Even though Jenny noticed small changes, there were many days she thought that for the amount of effort she was putting in she should be seeing bigger results. Those disempowering thoughts only slowed her progress down and depleted unnecessary energy points. That's why staying focused on your vision is paramount.

Stage 7:
Practice and Duplication

You have had past success in the area of health… whether it was releasing several pounds, feeling like a million dollars after a workout, or feeling at peace inside your mind. Being able to practice and duplicate that success long term is the focus of Stage Seven.

Success should not be a matter of luck and hit or miss, it should be a result of systemized, on-purpose actions focused on a specific result. You must be able to duplicate your success or it is not success, it is a one-hit wonder. In 1981, the band Soft Cell did a cover song called *Tainted Love*. This is a beautiful example of a one-hit wonder and the inability to duplicate success.

Everyone today knows the classic sound *"bink bink"* from the song… *"Tainted Love."* The song was a number-one hit in seventeen countries and went on to set a then-Guinness World Record for the longest consecutive stay on the U.S. Billboard Hot 100 chart of forty-three weeks. The problem was that the band could not duplicate their success formula. While they had some other hits popular in other countries, nothing came close to *Tainted Love*.

What's the difference between a one-hit wonder band and another who lasts for decades? If you look at bands that are wildly known and popular today like Aerosmith who began in 1970 or Bon Jovi who began in 1983, they have a formula for success and know how to duplicate it. This has allowed them to learn from their failures enough to survive several different generations of musical taste while other big bands from their generation are nothing but a memory. Those successful bands put most of their energy, most of the time, over a long period of time, into one focus—their music. What is the result when you duplicate success by having one focus over decades of time?

Aerosmith currently demands over one million dollars a show (lasting about three hours) and are still actively touring the world after almost *thirty-eight* years. Bon Jovi just released their tenth studio album as of the writing of this book. The album debuted at Number #1 on the Billboard charts and sold 292,000 copies in its first week on sale in the U.S. alone! After touring for almost a quarter of a century, their latest concert at a 23,000-seater stadium sold out within one minute of tickets being released.

Are you someone who complains about not seeing a result after exercising and eating better for three weeks, and then quits? What would happen if you did it consistently for thirty-eight years?

Example

Jenny definitely found this stage to be important, especially since she tended to yo-yo in the past with no means of duplicating any of her successes. When it came to health, it was not so much physical exercise or healthy eating that she had trouble with; it was more the health of her self-esteem and her beliefs. The biggest breakthrough for Jenny was understanding why she yo-yoed with her weight in the past so she would not practice that failing behavior anymore.

BEING FULFILLED

Jenny, like most people, tended to focus very externally when it came to her health. She focused on her body weight and vanity versus how she felt about herself on the inside. When she used fad diets and external "magic pills" like fat burners and other unregulated supplements, she achieved limited fulfillment. Therefore, the fulfillment she did have was not even the results of the hard work she put in. Hence, the results did nothing to improve her self-esteem and internal self-worth.

Jenny was reminded of the story of a friend who decided to have liposuction to lose weight and "tighten up." This woman had worked out for a few months and seen some results, but they were not quick enough for her. She was constantly depressed, and every time she looked in the mirror she would say, "I feel ugly."

All she wanted was a flat stomach and a tighter butt. After the procedure was complete and the bandages were ready to be taken off, she was very excited. The doctor carefully removed all the bandages and was very pleased. He said, "Go to the mirror and look at your new beautiful body!" She took a good look and was overwhelmed. She looked at her new flat stomach and tight butt and began to cry.

These tears, however, were not of joy; they were of sadness. To the surprise of the doctor, this woman was just as depressed as she was before surgery. Her body had changed on the outside, but it had remained the same on the inside. She did not do anything to deserve this body. Even though she physically saw something new, all she could see was the same ugly person she was before the surgery. When the doctor asked what was wrong, the woman replied, "I know I look different, but I still feel ugly."

What's Next?

At this point, revisit the questions at the beginning of this section and the definition you wrote for health fulfillment. See if you can answer any of the questions differently and more easily this time. Now that you have read through this section, continue on to the other sections. When finished, if you determine that health will be your main focus, come back to this section and go through all the stages and steps. Know that each stage will take some time to do, and there is no set time frame for them. Be patient and take it one step at a time.

The next section is dedicated to those career-driven business professionals and entrepreneurs who are focusing so diligently on creating greater financial wealth. If you want to create bigger bucks, you must know what comes first...

BEING FULFILLED

SECTION VI

BETTER BODY, BIGGER BUCKS

Many entrepreneurs and career driven business people with great intentions have sacrificed their health for their visions and passion. It becomes easy to put one's health and well-being on the back burner while striving for business success. This is true whether you are growing your own business or have a job. When you are on the go and traveling all the time, it's so easy to munch on convenient foods or forget to eat altogether. Most business owners are convinced that they cannot make time to work out and eat well. It's understandable. With the laser-like focus it requires to build a successful business, it's not a surprise that an entrepreneur's own health can move ten to fifteen places down on the priority list.

The major question you must ask yourself is: "What is this costing me?" Not in just health terms, but in your bottom-line profit. Even if you can honestly say, "I don't care about my health right now; I must focus on my business," think of it like this: focus on your business through your health.

Most business professionals that have recognized the importance of regular exercise and eating well have realized that they can't afford *not* to create the time to do these valuable activities. *Peak performance in business demands peak health and well-being.*

BEING FULFILLED

How profitable is your business? This is a common question that should be assessed regularly. What the majority of professionals fail to ask is: "How profitable is my body?" Whether you want to admit it or not, **your current level of health and well-being absolutely influences your profit margin.** At the end of the day, if you have a better physical and emotional body, you will earn bigger bucks... Better Body, Bigger Bucks!

As with any business decision, you deserve to take a look at how your lifestyle affects not only your own health, but also your bottom line. It does not matter how "well" you think you are doing, increasing your health will unequivocally increase your profits. There are plenty of professionals doing "well" by any standards that are in miserable health... by any standards.

Having coached many multiple, multiple millionaires whose health was no better than a smoldering cigarette, it was obvious how poor health inhibited their profits... even when they were generating multiple millions *a month!* The question becomes: What would be possible if their health improved significantly? Not only would they enjoy their profits more now, they would most certainly have the energy to create more, and better yet, be around to enjoy them in the future.

When you get strung out and burn both ends of the candle, you don't feel well. You don't have the energy to deal with your business, or even more importantly, with life. It's time to bring back structure into your life and take care of yourself so you can take care of the business. This way, you will have the physical and emotional wherewithal to do what is required. Your business will profit considerably from your general happiness and your ability to manage stress better.

SECTION VI – BETTER BODY, BIGGER BUCKS

There is something known in business called the trickle-down effect. This states that the behavior of a team, whether it be employees, downline, or coworkers, is a reflection of its leaders. Ultimately, the company's results trickle down from the top. Whether you are at the top or not, accept the responsibility that health begins with you... results begin with you. If you are healthy, your business will be healthy. There is a direct correlation.

The link between health and profits is not breaking news. Researchers have looked at whether staying healthy and fit can help your chances at succeeding in business. There have been studies done with commercial real estate stockbrokers. Those who had regular exercise routines earned significantly larger sales commissions than those that did not. Another study looked at employees from a plastic equipment company who exercised thirty to forty minutes, *at least* four times a week. Those workers showed significant improvement in productivity and job satisfaction compared with those who didn't. In fact, the largest percentage of that company's promotions went to the regular exercisers... Better Body, Bigger Bucks!

Take a look at the most wildly successful business people you know who model the unlimited wealth model. The majority of them have a regular exercise program. The Better Body part does not mean they look like a Victoria Secret model or like they belong on the cover of Gentleman's Quarterly. It means that they take care of themselves and are aware of bettering their health.

This does not mean that if you do not eat well or exercise you will not succeed in business. There are plenty of examples that prove that wrong. But in order to really see how profitable your business can be and to attain unlimited wealth, you absolutely must eat well and exercise. **In**

order to enjoy the fruits of your labor tomorrow, you must take care of yourself today.

Many entrepreneurs struggle with the thought that they are the face of their business. If they are not there constantly working it, there will be no income. Heck, many are constantly working it and there is still no income coming in! Even if you are established and have passive revenue streams, more likely than not you still feel like you must be there. What most highly successful entrepreneurs have experienced is that when they finally let go of having to "be there" all the time and finally begin taking care of themselves, their profits multiply significantly and they find themselves wondering where all the money was hiding. Prosperity will become effortless, and your bank account will reflect that.

Health Equity

Entrepreneurship is not always easy and neither is eating well or exercising. Entrepreneurs often live a lonely business life. We are in contact with customers, clients, employees, and our tax consultant, but oftentimes we are in the office alone and do not have a confidant for discussing new ideas, issues, or a difficult client. We are so buried in the business that we may lack a social outlet. This is where a place to vent, discuss, brainstorm, discover, and create new actions is important. In addition, having workout buddies or a training environment (like boot camp or group fitness classes) can provide a great venting place and sounding board keeping you fresh so you can continue producing. These groups will also assist you in exercise adherence.

While there are immediate payoffs for you and your business in adopting a healthy lifestyle, not all the benefits are so immediate. The choices you create today will affect the quality of your life in years to come. This mostly plays into your retirement years when you can really enjoy the fruits of your labor.

In a study published in *The Journal of the American Medical Association* in 2003, researchers estimated that the years of life lost due to obesity ranged from five to twenty, depending on gender and race. Five to twenty years! That tells only part of the story. Excess weight will also affect the number of disability-free years you enjoy. When you take into account physical quality of life, the effects of obesity are actually equivalent to thirty years of aging, according to research published in 2002 in the journal *Health Affairs*. That is insane!

Think about healthy living in economic terms. Let's say that each of us is endowed with a certain "stock of health." This stock either helps or hinders how much satisfaction we achieve over the course of our lives. An example would be a fit seventy-year-old retiree who travels, dances, and cycles while another is unable to walk long distances and live without medication. Who wants to live like that? That is called being dependent. We spend most of our younger years yearning to become independent... so our retirement should be the ultimate independence.

Ultimately, according to this economic theory, we weigh the perceived hassles of leading a healthy life today (comparing nutrition labels, for example) with our perceived payoff in the future. **If you don't put much value on your quality of life in the future, or simply don't give it much thought, then you will be less likely to do much about exercise and eating well now.**

What about your own economic model? Are you discounting the future value of your health as you age in order to avoid the perceived short-term inconveniences of activity and great nutrition?

Another component to this economic theory is viewing exercise and healthy eating as building equity. Take buying property, for example. Real estate is one of the most evident examples of how equity can pay off big time… long-term… and if you know what you are doing, it can pay very well in the short-term, too. Every dollar that you invest in your property will multiply significantly over a period of time. This does not even take effort; consistent monthly payments over twenty or thirty years will produce large equity in later life.

The same goes for exercise. Every minute you invest in your body will multiply significantly over time. Once again, this does not even take much effort; consistent weekly workouts at a good intensity over twenty or thirty years will produce a large health equity in later life.

Common Mindset

Why don't more people do this? First of all, most people don't think long-term; they do what is easier now versus what is more difficult now and more beneficial later. The second problem is that most people have a warped sense of what great health and nutrition are. Take a look at the images people compare themselves to and the diets that are on the market. These images and diets create unrealistic models.

SECTION VI – BETTER BODY, BIGGER BUCKS

Life as an entrepreneur poses some difficult odds to overcome. No one will give you a guarantee that your business will be successful. So if you are like most people, you do your best and take the plunge into the unknown. Every day, you roll up your sleeves, face down the odds, and dig in. You become stronger by educating yourself on what is out there and how you fit into that educated picture.

The mindset you must have to produce a profitable business is the mindset you will require for a healthy lifestyle as well. Going for a walk takes effort, and only you can create the decision to eat more fruits and vegetables. Just as in business, the odds of success can seem like a long shot. Research has found that fewer that twenty percent of the adults trying to reduce or maintain their weight were complying with the recommended guidelines on boosting physical activity and cutting calories.

I have seen this firsthand from investing twelve plus years as a personal trainer. If fewer than twenty percent are adhering to minimum guidelines, the rest are lying to themselves and pretending not to know. They keep saying, "But I am working so hard and eating well, and nothing is happening… I might as well quit."

The fact that less than twenty percent are complying with the guidelines set out to actually achieve a result is not surprising, yet telling. This is called struggling. Are you a struggleaholic? Day in and day out, are you struggling to lose weight or produce a result in your business, yet the whole time you are not really even doing what is required to actually produce that result? Do you keep telling yourself that you are working so hard, going to the gym eight days a week and working seventy hours a week, yet seeing no progress?

This is where the classic saying, "Work smarter, not harder" comes into play. The odds are that you could get one hundred percent better results in two days at the gym and thirty hours in the office if you took the time to get honest and educate yourself. Being serious about the Seven Stages and honoring your ten energy points each day will assist you to achieve better results.

Your Money *IS* Where Your Mouth Is

Put your money where your mouth is… Better yet, what goes into your mouth has a direct impact on your bottom line. Think about it like this: what you choose to eat is your *nutrition for bigger bucks!* Let me simplify nutrition for you: Input equals output. That's all you are required to know. In this case, the input is food and the output would be *not* how your body looks, but how well you perform in your business, how well your body functions to be able to produce a result.

Knowledge of nutrition is undervalued. This is because people think they know enough about it, and so they become incapable of learning. When you open up your mind, everything will change. Whatever level you are on, realize that nutritious fuel will impact your business *and your life* greatly. Great nutrition will keep you alert and alive versus sleepy and sluggish. It will maximize your performance and your income.

With literally thousands of fad diets and choices, the formula can seem complicated. Remember the commercial jingle, "You are what you eat from your head down to your feet?" Well, it's true. If you eat like crap, you'll feel like crap, and you'll perform like crap… and ultimately your bank account will look like crap, too.

There is a great method for identifying how your input (food) impacts your output (business performance). Keep a journal of how you feel throughout the day, in relation to your food intake. Generally ask questions like: "How do I feel twenty, forty and sixty minutes after eating?" After looking at how your input affects you, focus on your output. Generally ask questions like: "How am I sleeping? How did I feel before, during, or after my business presentation? How alert am I with clients?" That's the output.

From that information you will be better able to determine what fuel is right for you. This is the key—determine what fuel is right for YOU. Not what diet is right for YOU—what fuel is right for YOU. Not what fuel is right for everybody, but what FUEL is right for YOU.

When athletes perform well, they immediately ask themselves what they ate as early as a few days before the event, up to and including the foods they consumed during the event. Over time they can predict what foods work best for them specifically and what times are appropriate to eat them for maximal performance. Business is no different. Discover what foods to eat and the appropriate times to eat to keep you alert and high functioning during your business day. If an athlete takes so much consideration and planning on how to optimize their nutrition for a three-hour event, why shouldn't you be doing the same for a three-hour business event?

In the world of business, many people are tracking their performance. There are measures of performance that people, websites, machines, and marketing campaigns are comparing and tracking. The measure most overlooked is the performance derived from your nutrition. Do you ever feel sluggish during your day? Some people's solution is to take a nap during the day when they feel this way. How does that solution impact your bottom line? What is your solution when you get sluggish or crash energetically during your day? An extra-large Starbucks?

Many people attack the effect of feeling sluggish by masking it with a nap or a Starbucks. This is the same as a plumber fixing a leaky pipe by putting a piece of duct tape on it—a temporary solution at best! Nutrition for bigger bucks will allow you to discover the cause of your fatigue and subpar performance by identifying what foods caused the feeling.

Beyond the business skills you have developed, your business performance and ultimately your results rest on what you eat. While you can do well just from the great business skills you develop, huge profits are derived from taking a closer look at your input (food) and how it directly impacts your business output.

This takes work. Your initial thoughts might be: "I cannot take the time to look at my diet along with everything else; I just have to keep on working." I'm not talking about doing food journals and calorie counting, I'm simply asking you to be more conscious of:

1) what foods you are eating
2) when you are eating them
3) how you feel and ultimately perform after you eat them

You deserve to find great educators in the area of nutrition. Through their knowledge and inspiration, you can become much better at understanding how you can maximize your physical and mental energy via the foods you eat and the vitamins you supplement with. Please remember, even with much experience it can be difficult finding the "the best" multivitamins and foods that work for you. There is so much bogus information to sift through; however, when you do find "the best," the reward will be energy, love, power, money, fulfillment, and so much more.

Begin by asking the people you trust, the ones that are having the type of success you are seeking. Ask them how they did it and what they use. Constantly trying to reinvent the wheel and do it yourself it will be exhausting. Toss the thought that no one can do it better than you and model success just like you did in Stage One where you created a vision.

Most people are more than happy to share what they use and why. But please remember, just because it works for someone else, this does not mean it will work for you. At the end of the day, after you have given a process its due diligence, you must determine its value in *your* world. I could tell you flat out what vitamins to take, what foods to eat, or how to maximize your exercise program... but in the end, you must take the responsibility to see how those recommendations work for you.

What You Intuitively Know But Don't Want to Hear

"You can't judge a book by its cover." Yes, you can—people do it all the time. People are doing it to you right now. **Today, judgment is the engine of society, and we must accept that fact if we want to be successful.** In the world of business, judgment is one of the key influences that will drive a sale. A skilled salesperson or a well-developed marketing piece has the ability to sway judgment in order to close a sale.

Because of judgment, companies invest millions of dollars in branding, presentation, and market research to ensure that their "market" of potential customers perceive the look, image, and feel that particular company desires them to see. Using the wrong word or picture can portray the incorrect image and cost a company millions in revenue. Marketing and branding is a place where simple intuition and relying on a gut feeling will not work and can cost a fortune in lost profits.

A great example of this is a story from the book, *Mindless Eating.* The author, Brian Wansink, was working on a consulting project for *Better Homes and Gardens Magazine* (BH&G). One day the director of editorial research showed him four different BH&G cover ideas for an issue that was being published in ten months. All four had the same cover photo and looked identical when he first saw them from four feet away. When he moved closer, he discovered the only thing that differed were the six "cover blurbs," or teaser phrases, on the left side of the cover.

The director asked Brian to predict which cover would sell the most copies and why. Brian pointed to one and said, "I think this one will do the best because it uses shorter little phrases." Without blinking, the director said, "Your intuition just cost us over one million dollars in newsstand sales." The director went on to explain that every month BH&G took the best ideas for cover stories, developed four or more sample covers with a different mix of blurbs, and then asked over a thousand nonsubscribers which version they would be most likely to buy off the newsstand. With a circulation base of over 7.2 million readers, BH&G did not use hunches and intuition. They did research so they could predict which magazine a blonde, thirty-seven-year-old mother of two in Wisconsin would pick up, flip through, and buy when standing in the checkout line at Safeway.

While effective marketing and branding from a company's perspective is very purposeful, from a consumer's perspective it is very emotional and intuitive. That's why it is your job to be consciously aware of the words you speak and the vision you portray... this is the brand "You." There is great energy around images and words. Take a look at how "labels" are changing today. A stewardess is now called a flight attendant. Gyms are now being called health clubs because gyms were for muscle heads and can be intimidating.

Having spoken in health clubs across the US and Canada since 1998, I have seen firsthand how marketing and new member presentations have changed. Today's public is judgmental and more skeptical than ever, mostly because they are looking for a good reason not to do what they perceive to be painful (working hard at something without the guarantee of a result).

BEING FULFILLED

As a business entrepreneur, you must be keenly aware that *you* are the product; *you* are the brand. *People will decide on your product, service, or business and even pay more than your competitor charges simply because they like you!* The bottom line: **you will be judged for your appearance and how you look.** Deeper than that, *people will judge the energy that you send out when they interact with you.*

First impressions *are* lasting… you'd better believe it. When you are feeling tired and sluggish, you cannot mask that tired energy. All the coffee and cosmetics in the world cannot mask energy. Remember that in Philosophy #4: Results are Energy we outlined how energy cannot lie. Your nutrition determines how you feel and the energy you transmit. Your level of physical and emotional fitness also determines how you feel and the energy you transmit. These will play a huge role in whether you close the sale or not.

Example: Would you buy a high definition television from a blind person? Would you buy a Mercedes from a car dealer who just stepped out of their Lexus? Would you hire a personal trainer who was obese? No. Why? It is counterintuitive; it goes against what you feel should be right. In the world of judgment, these people *at a glance* are not walking the walk. They will have to work a hundred times harder than someone that does fit the intuitive profile of the product or service they represent. You do not write the rules; just make sure that you understand and follow them, and you will magnify your success.

If you are having trouble accepting this… stop trying to be nice. This is not about being nice. "Nice" will not allow you the results you are looking to create. If you are overweight, for example, and represent a fitness or nutritional product, the fact is that you will have a more difficult time being successful than your fit counterpart... all skills being equal. This does not mean you cannot be successful; it just means the odds are not in your favor. As it is, the odds are not in anyone's favor, so why create a more difficult situation?

"But Jeff, it is not easy." "But Jeff, I have a situation or condition." I can appreciate that. But the bottom line is: **the customer does not care.** They want the most value for their investment. In the majority of sales, a large part of their value comes from you.

I was a personal trainer for twelve years before retiring. I worked with some trainers over the years that were less than fit "looking." "Looking" is the key word. They looked like the average person, yet they were fitter than most. That "look" was a component that held them back from having a super large clientele. Is that fair? Heck no, they were great trainers, but life is not fair. Swallow that fact.

When I was doing personal training, I would always ask the people who hired me their reasons for doing so. Inevitably, one of the answers in the top three was that I was in great shape. In my twelve years as a personal trainer, I was *never* asked how many certifications I had or if I had references. People hired me for three reasons: 1) I was super fit; 2) My clients had fun with me; 3) They loved my energy. The word result is not even in there! Yes, I achieved incredible results with people, but that was not the top reason people hired me. To this day as a coach, people will hire me for the same reasons. It is an attractive energy that people want to be around and want more of. It is physical, emotional, and spiritual vibrancy!

When you emit this vibrancy, you will almost never get asked where you went to school, how many degrees you have, how long you have been doing something, how successful you are, how much money you make, or how old you are. The logical, analytical thinker might ask no matter what, but even they will be attracted to what you possess without much need for details. Those details are the "statistics" of your résumé. For true fulfillment, become aware of your energetic résumé and what it sends out. All skills aside, this energetic résumé will carry the most weight in your business success and ultimately close the sale for you.

Coach's Challenge

The main role of a great coach is to objectively listen and ask great, probing questions that allow for discovery and lead to results. This challenge is all about questions. The following questions are specifically designed to enhance your understanding of the material just presented on the brand "You." Some questions are from live coaching sessions that have uncovered amazing answers.

Answer each group of questions in order.

Group One: *Recognizing Your Brand*

- *If I were a product in a supermarket, where would I be located and what would I be?*
- *Would I have a label? If so, what would it read?*
- *If I checked out my nutrition label, what would I see? (Use Figure G)*
- *If I looked at my ingredients, what would the first three be? (Use Figure G)*

- *Describe the person who most frequently puts you in their shopping cart. Include what this person would look like physically, how they earn money, and how much they earn.   Be as specific and detailed as possible.*
- *Would you buy you? Why or why not?*
- *What have you learned about your answers to these questions that can assist you in improving your results in business and health?*
- *How specifically will you implement putting these lessons into action?*

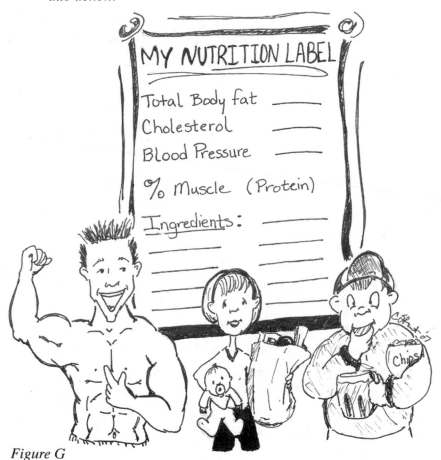

Figure G

BEING FULFILLED

Group Two: *Your Business-Fitness Connection*

- *Look back over the previous twelve months. Honestly, how was your health? Describe in great detail, using specifics.*
- *If you were to rate your health this past year on a scale of one to ten, ten being the best and one the worst, what would it be?*
- *Look back over the previous twelve months. Honestly, how profitable was your business? Describe in great detail, using specifics.*
- *If you were to rate your business profits this past year on a scale of one to ten, ten being the best and one the worst, what would it be?*
- *Based on the above answers and ratings, what connection or common themes can you see between your level of health and your business profit for the past twelve months? Describe this in great detail.*
- *How has your level of health over the past twelve months directly impacted your business this past year, for good or bad? Be specific.*
- *Based on your specific findings, what are two specific areas you are committed to improving over the next twelve months?*
- *What's your motivation for improving these areas?*
- *If you have ever tried to improve these areas in the past, why is this time different?*
- *What is your plan to move forward and who will assist you?*

Group Three: *Your Better Body, Bigger Bucks*

- *What are the habits of a person who owns a million-dollar body? If you don't know, just give it a go or ask someone. You can begin by writing: A person who has a million-dollar body does "____" on a daily basis. (Please know that a million-dollar body is not a big-breasted, six-pack, tight butt model on the cover of a magazine. It is what you require to feel fulfilled)*

- *Identify what habits you currently express that result in the health you have today. Be specific and detailed. Compare your habits to the ones you wrote above*

- *Based on the comparison, what is one new habit you would like to create over the next several months? (Refer to Philosophy #2 on how to create a new habit.)*

- *What are the habits of a person who owns a million-dollar bank account? If you don't know, just give it a go or ask someone. You can begin by writing: A person who has a million-dollar bank account does "____" on a daily basis. (Please know that a million dollar bank account does not have to have millions in it. It is what you require to feel fulfilled)*

- *Identify what habits you currently express that earn you the income you have today. Be specific and detailed.*

- *Based on the comparison, what is one new habit you would like to create over the next several months? (Refer to Philosophy #2 on how to create a new habit.)*

Your Path to a Better Body
and Bigger Bucks:
"Jeff's Experiment"

Hopefully answering the questions from group three in the Coach's Challenge have assisted you in discovering what a million-dollar body and bank account means to you. The following material is designed to assist you in bringing those visions and habits into reality via empowering feelings.

I have achieved an extreme level of fitness at different points of my life, and I maintain a strong level now. Financially, I have achieved an income that puts me in the top five percent of society, and even though it is not a million-dollar bank account yet, I am well on the way. That being said, I wanted to see the connection of what it feels like at each of these extreme levels of fitness and income... so I did a little "experiment."

I don't know what a million-dollar bank account feels like, but I do know what a million-dollar body feels like. So I wrote down all the feelings of having a million-dollar body:

Empowering	*Amazing*
Sexy	*Strong*
Invincible	*Fulfilled*
Secure	*Fun*

Then I was really curious, and I wondered what a million-dollar bank account feels like. So I asked some of the millionaire friends and clients I have what a million-dollar bank account feels like. Can you guess what I found? Exactly! The feelings from both lists were strikingly similar. In fact, for each of the feelings I wrote in my list, I found at least three of them in every millionaire's list! The best part... one millionaire wrote down sexy! Sexy... how stinkin' cool is that? A million dollar bank account feels sexy! I am all over that.

Here's why I did this. I know that I have the potential to be a millionaire and am on that path. My only setback in the past was that having an income of $83,000 or more per month was unfathomable for me at one time (as it is for most people). When you are earning five, ten or even thirty thousand a month, eighty or more might seem impossible. This feeling of impossibility is the same when it comes to achieving a seven-figure body. If you are thirty pounds overweight and cannot see your feet because your stomach is in the way, a six-pack might seem impossible.

I see this struggle all the time when I coach entrepreneurs as well as people at my health club. The entrepreneurs are romancing the potential of earning thirty, fifty, and one hundred thousand a month. The health club people are romancing six-pack abs and defined arms. In the end, most are left defeated and end up quitting. The purpose here is to create a situation where you know you can achieve this larger income and or healthier body without the overwhelmed feelings. Here is how.

After I discovered that having a million-dollar body feels just like having a million-dollar bank account, I was thrilled. My excitement was so high because I recognize the power of attractive energy and how like attracts like. This is why I presented these topics of attraction and energy to you already in Philosophy #4: Results are Energy. I know that I don't have to have, in reality, a million-dollar bank account to know what it feels like. But by knowing how what I want feels like, I can focus on situations that allow me to feel that way now.

By consciously choosing to feel this way on a consistent basis, I will emit that vibrant energy I spoke of earlier and attract the people necessary for my fulfillment. My mentor and coach, Jeffrey Combs, always told me that I was one or two contacts away from a multiple six- or seven-figure income. I did not fully understand what he meant until I learned the above principles and attracted those people into my life.

If you don't have a million-dollar bank account *or* body, and you're seeking to achieve them, that's okay, you don't require either to begin. Look at an area where you have felt similar feelings like the ones I listed before. I guarantee you too know what it feels like to have the type of fulfillment you are seeking mainly because *you have already experienced those feelings* in other areas. Once you determine when you had those feelings, you can use them in the present to leverage your fulfillment. Goals are really feelings, and you can experience those feelings any time you want simply by shifting your focus. Focus = Feel.

When you leverage these feelings into the present and live them daily, you begin to attract the people and situations necessary for your desired fulfillment. Besides, at the end of the day, we have all physically and emotionally felt really great at some point. When you had those feelings of being healthy and fit, what did you feel like? Like a million dollars! So don't tell yourself you don't know what it feels like to have a million-dollar body or bank account. *The following coach's challenge will assist you with understanding how to create better results right now using your feelings.*

Coach's Challenge

This purpose of this challenge is to expand upon the last paragraph where you learned that goals are really feelings and you can experience those feeling any time you want simply by shifting your focus. It is paramount that you experience this challenge to enhance your odds of success and fulfillment.

1. Write down one goal that you want to achieve. Let's not make this the grand goal of your life, but something achievable in six months or so.

Keep it simple._____

_____

_____

_____

2. Write down the feeling(s) you will have when you achieve that goal. Example: alive, energetic, sexy, fulfilled, or powerful.

_____

3. Write down when you will achieve the goal. Day, month, time—just pick when.

Now, read out loud what you wrote for your goal. Out loud!

Which number did you read out loud as your goal? Did you read what you wrote down for number one? Great... but that is not your goal! Number one is never your goal; number one is just a strategy to achieve number two. THAT IS YOUR GOAL... number two!

Why number two? When we set out to do something, what we really want is the feeling we experience (#2) when we accomplish the strategy (#1). The wonderful part about this is that you can choose to create that feeling (#2) anytime you want to have it! Creating the desired feeling is simply a matter of shifting your focus to a thought that will allow you to feel what you want. I call this Focus = Feel.

When you focus on something, you will experience it via a feeling. Once you have shifted your feeling to a desirable one, you are more likely to create action versus procrastinate. Bottom line: **Goals are really feelings.** There is an incredible exercise on how to shift your focus to feel differently on my 8-CD audio course *Healthy Mind, Healthy Body.* (See back of book in the resource section)

Let's put into writing what you wrote down earlier so you can better see this new perspective.

My goal is to feel (#2)_____

My strategy to feel that way is (#1)_____

Now, what energetic message does what you wrote for number three send to you? It says that you are putting those feelings from number two in the future, and you are not allowing yourself to feel them in the present. What are you doing by denying yourself that feeling? How does that affect your daily progress? How about allowing yourself to experience the feelings of number two and taking action right now? That will help you accomplish what you are setting out to do. You can have that feeling anytime; it does not have to be attached to a strategy or a time frame.

Denying yourself a feeling that you want to feel because you think it is tied to a strategy or a time frame is a source of procrastination. If you think about it, we give ourselves the feelings that we experience on a moment-by-moment basis. We decide how we are going to feel, and then we live into it. Example: What is an excuse you have used before *not* to exercise? People use the "I'm too tired" excuse a lot. Once you tell yourself that you are too tired, you believe it. You decide that you are too tired to work out, and you live into it by rationalizing and believing your own excuse! You keep looking for reasons why you are tired to further prove how you decided you were feeling. What happens to your goals when you decide on feeling tired?

Here is how you can use this new perspective that goals are really feelings. Imagine what would happen if EVERY morning you woke up and *decided* to feel what you wrote for number two? Remember Philosophy #3: Fulfillment Is a Conscious Choice. No more excuses in thinking about the strategy or time frame, but rather allow yourself to feel your goal every day. Raise your hand if you feel you would create better odds of achieving your goals by doing this! Like the Bon Jovi song, *Raise Your Hands!* Straight from the song he sings:

> *"Raise your hands… when you wanna let it go*
> *Raise your hands… when you wanna let a feeling show!"*

Beer-Gut Mentality

Teaching yourself to feel great on all levels is a very important first step. This is called emotional fitness… where we have a command of our emotions. It is not control, or power; it is simply an understanding of why our emotions are there and what they represent—a signal, if you will. After this awareness, **creating new behaviors that form great habits will be the key factor** in actually achieving your dream in the real world. Reference Philosophy #2: Great Habits Produce Great Results.

Who is at the health club consistently? Someone with habits. Who is at the health club in the middle of July? Someone with *great* habits (or an addiction!). Are you trying to build a fit and healthy body on a sedentary lifestyle habit? Are you trying to build a flat stomach with a beer-gut mentality? That's the same as trying to earn a six-figure income on fifty-thousand-dollar habits. A fifty-thousand-dollar habit will produce fifty-thousand-dollars. A beer-gut mindset will produce a beer gut. It is the same as what you get when you squeeze lemons.

Is your body for profit? Is your business for profit? The habits of a nonprofit body will result in a nonprofit business and vice versa. It can be seen as a two-way street, because the feelings are so similar. In the end, you get paid for how you feel. The heath of your mind and body can determine the size of your paycheck. And the size of your paycheck can determine the health of your mind and body. Because they both have significant influence over each other, it is important to grasp the connection between business and fitness. By doing so, you will not only be able to achieve better fitness results, but also reduce stress, increase sales, create effective business management systems, use them to find unique networking opportunities, and become a leader at home as well as at work. Ultimately, you will create a more profitable business and feel fulfilled.

What's Next?

Now that you know creating a better physical and emotional body leads to bigger bucks, the next section takes a fresh and very unique approach to creating better health results in your life.

BEING FULFILLED

SECTION VII

MULTIPLE STREAMS
OF FITNESS

What does it take to create the bank account you dream of? Many factors influence this, including having multiple streams of income. This concept was presented earlier and defined as creating profit with money coming in from multiple sources. If you have only one stream of income, like a job, and you are laid off, your bank account dries up.

This concept is absolutely the best way to truly create huge profits. Whether your profits come from multiple businesses or different products and services in one business, having multiple streams of income allows you the freedom to benefit from all sources versus "putting all your eggs in one basket."

This concept is also prevalent in the investing world. Most people investing in the market today have a diversified portfolio. If you have 100% of your monies in one company and something happens to that company… you get the point.

When a concept works well in one area, it can also be applied successfully to another area because basic human behavior patters replicate in all areas of our lives. Because we have a tendency to replicate behavior patterns in all areas of our lives, it is important to recognize *what* behavior patterns we are replicating. Do you replicate success patterns or failure patterns? Business, relationships, and health all have a direct link in that the behaviors and habits it takes to be fulfilled in each are very similar.

So, if you can create vast riches in business with multiple streams of income, you should be able to produce vast riches in health via *multiple streams of fitness*. Fitness is a world that very few people understand. This includes people in the fitness profession, too. People tend to complicate a very simple process, just like in business. Business is a simple process once you understand some laws and philosophies and begin to consistently apply them over time. *The purpose of this section is to simplify the process of fitness to increase your odds of success and apply that understanding to other areas of your life to become fulfilled.*

> **An important note:** Don't confuse simple with easy. Success in fitness is simple yet not easy to attain. There are simple concepts and actions to take; however, the work is not necessarily easy. For example, riding a bike is simple. Riding a bike trying to keep up with Lance Armstrong is not easy. Picking up the phone and creating a call is simple. Connecting and closing the sale is something completely different. Both require extensive training and consistent practice over a long period of time to achieve the desired result.

Dive into the Lake of Fitness

It is time to define Multiple Streams of Fitness. Imagine your level of fitness as a huge lake you are swimming in with multiple streams flowing in and out. There is an optimal level of water that this lake should be at. If it is too high it will flood; if it's too low, it will be dry. In order for the lake to remain at this optimal level, there must be an overall balance of the water coming in and leaving. There are times when it rains heavily or the snow melts and the water level is too high. There are also times when it has been very dry out, and the water level drops.

Your level of fitness is no different. Because there is so much that goes into defining fitness, for simplicity sake, fitness in this model refers to as your body weight. Your body weight, like the water in the lake, has an optimal level. When your body weight is too high, you are overweight; too low, you are gaunt looking. The multiple streams that are coming in and out of your fitness lake determine your level of fitness. Think of the multiple streams as input and output.

Input: *This is what you put into your body (calories); it's what goes into the lake. We will label this as Multiple Streams of Nutrition.*

Output: *This is how you utilize that input; it's what goes out of the lake. We will label this as Multiple Streams of Exercise.*

Optimal Body Weight Redefined

Optimal body weight is NOT based on height and weight charts, contrary to what most people think. Do you base what you should be earning on average household income charts? Then you would be earning about $35,600 a year. If you don't do it with income, why do you do it with your weight?

True *optimal body weight is based on how you feel.* Here is the problem: People have been taught to measure their weight on a scale! Use a scale to measure deli meat or to see how much that fish you just caught weighs... but don't use a scale to tell you how you feel.

In my career as a personal trainer, I cannot tell you how many people worked so hard for so long. They would invest thousands of dollars, release tons of weight, drop countless pant sizes, and get hundreds of compliments while feeling on top of the world. Then they would step on a scale, and the number did not read what they wanted or expected. Based on a previous, society-inflicted negative connection with a number, they allowed that number to gut all that hard work and the great feelings they earned.

> In fitness, what are you listening to… a scale or your feelings?
>
> **Fulfillment comes when you ignore the external messages and trust the internal messages.**
>
> In this example, the external message is a number; the internal message is a feeling.

Multiple Streams of Nutrition

This is simply defined as the food you put into your body, or using our example, the water that flows into your lake of fitness. Have you ever been swimming in a lake that was very dirty and polluted? What causes a lake to become polluted? What nature and people throw into the lake determines its beauty and health. Your body is no different. What you put into your body will *absolutely* determine how you feel and ultimately look. That statement is not rocket science; however, isn't that the point? If it is indeed that simple, what is the problem of over 95 percent of the population who pollutes their body day after day?

The concept of multiple streams of nutrition will assist you in simplifying what you should and should not be eating. Without doing too much writing or thinking, if you were to mentally review your daily eating habits, you can get a clear picture of what these "multiple streams" look like. Anytime you put something in your mouth, ask yourself out loud: "What will this food do to my lake of fitness… pollute or beautify it?"

The answer is intuitively simple and logically difficult. In other words, if you listen to your heart, you will easily know what to do. If you listen to reason and logic, you will confuse yourself and be more likely to sell yourself a nice excuse. **Excuses reside in your logic; answers reside in your heart.**

The health and fitness industry has WAY overcomplicated nutrition... precipitated by a demand from the population. The population sends a message that says: "We do not have any time or will power and we need a quick fix." The fitness industry responds by producing thousands of products, services, and diets that confuse the population. This process fattens America as it fattens the fitness industry's wallets. The market is now saturated with information that is packaged well and marketed effectively, but which has left the average consumer frustrated and hopeless. The average person points the finger but does not realize that they are the cause.

I want to present you with a simple formula for eating well. For this to work, you must strip yourself from everything you have ever heard, read, or experienced about nutrition and eating well. Just for a moment, if you will, release the pressure that society and you have visited upon yourself. This will not work unless you put down all your rules and circumstances for a moment.

How to eat well: At the end of each day ask yourself this question. Which of these three numbers describes how I feel based on how I ate today?

1) Miserable; I overate
2) Average; I ate okay
3) Excellent; I ate really well

You must answer this question from the reference point of honesty and no rules. Simply go with how you feel. Based on your answer, in a given week, five or more days should be at a three: "Excellent; I ate really well." When you do this for three to five years in a row, you will be in significantly better health. If that seems too long for you, you are missing the big picture.

You can have an occasional "Miserable; I overate" day, but keep these to a minimum. If you think this is too difficult, you are right; it is difficult. If it were easy, then everyone would be doing it, and this book would not be necessary. Remember, this is a simple process, yet it can be a difficult journey. The good news: once you build the proper habits, it will become easier.

Most people will have a tendency to overanalyze what you just read. They will have all these "buts" and questions to clarify that dilute the simple process of the question: How well did you eat—poor, average, or great? Is that you? Are you resisting? Do you feel the need to question and clarify what was written? How does questioning and needing to know everything slow you down with your business, relationships, and health results? Why does eating a nutritious, well-balanced meal have to be so complicated? Why do *you* complicate it? What does that complication protect you from? How does all that research, reading, calorie counting, nutritional label reading and recording keep you safe from the truth? What is the truth? What is the real cause of your current result? Finally, congratulations if you have a handle on your nutrition.

When it comes to creating healthier food choices, quit creating excuses for the types of food you like to eat. Bacon, for example, does not constitute a healthy food. Have you told yourself: "I only have it when I eat out," or "This piece does not look too fatty." Most people love foods that are greasy and have "heart attack" written all over them. I'm not suggesting that you never have them again, but rather cut the lies and expose what choices you are creating that form your current results. You can still eat well and have ice cream and chips during your day. The difference is how much you eat and how frequently you eat them. Lots of "bad" foods don't result in "bad" results—lots of "bad" choices result in "bad" results.

The Energy of Nutrition

This energy is not the physical energy you receive from eating a bowl of pasta and then running thirteen miles. This is emotional energy that is wrapped up in the ease or stress *you create* from eating foods. The energy of nutrition is the signal that you transmit to the universe stemming from your relationship with food. This energy is directly connected to Philosophy #4: Results are Energy. When you wish to connect with people via the law of attraction, you will begin to recognize how important the energy of nutrition is.

When you have a great relationship with food and have "figured out" your nutrition, life will be simpler, and your path to unlimited wealth will come easier. You will be sending out a signal of ease, focus, and clarity to the universe. What type of person will be attracted to that? On the other hand, if eating is a daily stressor for you, that stress will negatively impact your results in business, relationships, and health. You will be sending out a signal of confusion, chaos, and frustration. What type of person will be attracted to that?

When you consistently eat poorly, you are living a contradiction. You have a desire to send a signal to yourself and the world of looking and feeling healthy, yet your actions are directly contradicting that. What messages are you sending to yourself while standing in front of the refrigerator at ten in the evening, not even hungry yet trying to convince yourself you are? What messages are you sending when you pretend to eat well in front of everyone, but when the house is empty you go for the stash of chocolate?

Talk about the biggest contradiction in the universe when you are literally stuffing food down your throat while all you can think about is how badly you feel now and how guilty you will feel when you're done. And all the while, you are on a fitness program and brand new diet. If you connect with any of this, revisit Stage 4 from the Seven Stages Applied to Health section under ContrAddiction. This will assist you on overcoming this pattern.

Multiple Streams of Exercise

Remember that your "lake of fitness" has an input and output. You just learned how the input of nutrition plays a role in your results. Now let's focus on your output, which is exercise. Multiple Streams of Exercise is the output that keeps the water level balanced in your lake. No matter who you are, or how well you eat, if you do not have at least one stream of exercise in your life, your lake will flood at some point. In other words, you will gain weight.

Eating well is an important component and cannot be overlooked. Exercise, however, is a much larger component to your overall feeling of well-being and fulfillment. While it is great to have an activity such as walking that you do for exercise, the concept here is to add multiple streams of exercise into your daily activity. If you love to walk outside and it is pouring rain or twenty below out, now what do you do? The excuse at that point actually becomes a valid reason. Having multiple streams of exercise will provide another avenue to exercise.

The goal is to create daily or even hourly situations where you are exercising. This does not mean hopping on your bike and hammering out fifty miles. This is a reminder of something you already know, but it's giving you a unique perspective on it so you might actually implement it. Has someone ever told you to take the stairs versus the elevator? What about parking at the end of the parking lot furthest from the door to walk a bit more? You have heard this, but who actually does it? These familiar strategies are what I call multiple streams of exercise.

Let's look at Cathy as an example. Her main focus is business, yet she realizes she requires exercise to stay healthy. In a typical week, her uncompromisable exercise time set up from the seven stages consists of two strength-training workouts and one bike ride. That is her consistent, scheduled exercise time when her intensity is through the roof. She realizes that to maintain the type of fitness she has achieved, she requires more than those three sessions. Because she only has so much energy each day, and it is mostly directed to her business, she must be creative in the ways she attains her fitness results. Let's take a glimpse of what Cathy does to ensure she has multiple streams of exercise in her day.

When Cathy sits in her home office writing, she requires breaks to stretch and refocus. When she takes a break, she will get down on the floor and do fifty or one hundred pushups, broken into as many sets as necessary.

Randomly throughout her day in between clients, she will also do quick sets of pushups, dips, abdominal work, and stretches. Sometimes she will sit on the floor and stretch while she is on the phone with a client. She *does* park on the far side of the parking lot, and she takes the stairs whenever possible. When she takes her dog out, she'll throw the ball around and chase him, which spikes her heart rate. Most of the time, this only takes five minutes. There are days when she does that five times, which is like doing a twenty-five-minute interval workout!

In the mornings before she goes into her office, she will take her dog and son for a ten- to twenty-minute walk up and down her hill. She also may hook up the bike trailer to her bike and go for a quick three-mile loop, pulling her son while her dog runs next to them. If Cathy is on the phone with an unimportant call or simply taking the laundry upstairs, she may go up and down the stairs six to ten times just to get her heart rate up. When she plays with her son, she uses him as resistance and does shoulder presses, bench presses, squats, lunges, and dips with him on her lap. He loves it, and she certainly works hard. When she sits in her Jacuzzi to relax or brainstorm, she always stretches her muscles.

Hopefully you can see the long-term benefits and health equity created by doing this. The question is: Will *you* do something like this? Statistically, about twenty percent who read this will do it for one to ten days before stopping. Five percent will do it for a longer period of time, maybe six months or five years. They will be fairly consistent, but not at the level to see the results they truly want. About one out of one hundred people will adopt this concept and utilize it to the maximum. Are you that one person?

Statistically, ninety-plus percent of the population does not stay in an activity long enough to reap the true results they desire, because they quit before it happens. In fact, the majority of great results are simply one or two steps away after you quit. The concept of Multiple Streams of Exercise is presented here so you can decide if it works for you. If you truly cannot find a larger block of time to become healthier, this concept works well.

What if you knew you were one workout away from feeling the way you want… one contact away from the large paycheck… one thought away from fulfillment? Would you stick it out, take the plunge, go another round? Attaining unlimited wealth and *being fulfilled* is not a matter of luck, karma, or prayer… it is conscious choice. Looking and feeling the way you dream of is a conscious choice. Creating the income that you desire is a conscious choice. Creating the relationship of your dreams is a conscious choice. Consciously choosing to put this book down and do as many pushups as you can *RIGHT NOW* is your conscious choice! Will you do it?

Residual Muscle Income

One of the best ways to earn money is by way of residual income, which is defined as working once and getting paid multiple times on that one effort. This is different from a job where you work an hour and get paid for that hour. In a job where you work once and get paid once, the odds of creating riches so that you can live out your dreams and retire large are slim to none. It is possible if you start young, save diligently, and create smart buying decisions throughout your life. But the fact is, most people don't.

There are so many ways in business that you can create a residual income, it is exciting. If you are willing to stay in the game long enough for your results to multiply, you will be more than set. Wouldn't it be nice to be able to take the concept of residual income and apply it to exercise? In other words, exercise once and get ongoing results from that one effort? Great news… you can with **Residual** Muscle **Income**.

Muscle is the major source of burning calories in your body, because muscle is metabolically active. This means that just to stay alive and operate properly, muscle is in constant need of calories. Think of muscle as a car that is idling all day and night… it's an engine that never shuts off. It's consuming fuel even while it is just sitting there. This is what your muscle does. When you use your muscles, you use more fuel—just like when you drive your car, you use more fuel. How much fuel you use depends on how hard you drive the muscle or car.

Have you ever heard the term "muscle car?" This defines a car that has a lot of horsepower and can really move. Would you say that car is fuel-efficient? Absolutely not… and we don't want our muscles to be fuel-efficient either, unless we are athletes, because that means they will burn lots of calories!

As you develop muscle, it grows. Think of it as having a bigger engine in a car. A bigger engine will consume more fuel than a smaller one. A bigger muscle will consume more energy (calories) than a smaller one. You might be thinking now, "But I don't want big muscles." If it makes you feel any better, call muscle lean body mass.

BEING FULFILLED

> I cannot tell you how many people I have encountered during my years as a fitness professional, both men and women, who say, "I don't want to bulk up or look like a bodybuilder. You won't! *It just will not happen!* If you *were* to work out and eat at the level *necessary* to look like that, you would not only feel more incredible than you could even imagine, but you would be very satisfied with the desired outcome.

Here is how you can benefit from residual muscle income. One pound of muscle burns about fifty calories a day. Let's say you begin a strength-training program and lift weights for a period of time. In that time, let's say you develop ten new pounds of muscle. Based on the figure above, you now would be burning an extra five hundred calories *a day* more than if you did not develop that muscle. (50 calories x 10 pounds of muscle = 500 calories a day)

The best part is that whether you work out or not in a given day, you will still burn that five hundred calories because your new ten pounds of muscle is still there, and it requires fuel! Just to give you a comparison, in order to burn five hundred calories each day in a cardiovascular workout such as running or biking, you would have to workout at least an hour at a moderate intensity. Do you have that type of time *every day?*

This is why *residual income* is so appealing, because whether you go to work or not, you still get paid! Even though you can choose to work or not in your residual income business on any given day, you know that if you leave it completely and never work it again, the proceeds, generally speaking, will decrease over time. The same goes for muscle. Don't expect to work out for six months, gain ten pounds of muscle, never lift a weight again, and expect the residual benefits to last forever.

With both business and health there can be a lot of up-front work when you do not get paid or see results. It can seem like you invest countless hours, even years, and not see the big results. The one who stays in the game longest will reap the biggest reward. Imagine creating a residual income stream that produced five hundred dollars *a day* on top of what you already produce. No matter what you currently earn; an extra $15,000 a month or $180,000 a year can never hurt. In the same way, developing ten pounds of muscle and burning five hundred calories a day adds up, too. Generally speaking, those 500 calories a day adds up to burning an extra 15,000 calories a month and the equivalent of burning fifty-one pounds of fat per year!

Proof that muscle truly is a calorie consumer can be seen in the different speeds men and women release weight. Besides the well-known fact that men are smarter than women, increased muscle mass is why men can release fat faster than women. Men simply have more muscle mass than women and can build it easier because of their testosterone levels.

The lowest optimal and healthy body fat percentage for a male is three percent compared to a female which is twelve percent. Ladies, have you ever gone on a diet with your husband or boyfriend? They stopped eating one thing, worked out a couple times a week, and lost twenty-five pounds. You gave up every food you love, hit the gym hard every day, and barely lost five pounds. Now you know why! Whoever you are, stop blaming and pick up some weights to create your **Residual** Muscle **Income.**

If You Are Easily Offended, Don't Read This

Here is where we get even more honest. When you are honest with yourself, you will not get offended. The following is undeniably true, and with the knowledge that we possess in today's world, it should not be ignored. The objective is to assist you in understanding the messages you are sending to the universe and more importantly to yourself via what you do or do not do. I will use smoking and fitness as examples.

Are you a smoker or nonsmoker? Are you an active or sedentary person? Whatever category you *choose* to be in, you must understand the messages that other people receive from you and they way they may judge you. If you smoke, what are you saying to the world and to yourself? Read the label off a cigarette box: "Warning: Smoking *causes* lung cancer, heart disease, emphysema, and complicates pregnancy." The box is literally saying: **You WILL die prematurely from smoking these,** and everyone intuitively knows this.

The warning label use to say "may cause" and now it says "causes." We know, you know, and they know, yet people still do it. What would you think if you walked past a young mom pushing her newborn baby while taking a nice drag on her cigarette? What she most likely does not realize is the message she is sending to the world, her baby, and herself.

It is the same with exercise. We know the amazing benefits that exercise provides physically, mentally, spiritually, and emotionally. There is no denying it. Yet the majority of the population does not exercise *at all*. Not exercising shortens your life and diminishes its quality just as smoking does. **With the evidence we have today, not exercising is the same as smoking a pack of cigarettes a day!**

This is not an attempt to shock you into working out or to quit smoking; that is your choice. The bigger picture is to show the energy of your action, which is what ultimately attracts your results. What you do or don't do creates a statement. What is the statement you create by not exercising? "I am consciously choosing to reduce the overall quality of my life." "I am choosing to decrease my potential as a human being in business and relationships, because I do not exercise."

With what we know today, if you do not exercise you are sending an unmistakable signal to *yourself* and the world that you don't care. How can anyone deny this? There is not an excuse big enough not to have some form of weekly exercise in your life. The problem is that most people have a big enough reason to have a weekly excuse in their life.

No matter what your physical and emotional condition, there is something you can do. A client of mine was a paraplegic who could only move from above the neck. He had breathing exercises he did daily to keep his lung capacity strong. He consistently did daily, specific exercises for his mind to keep it sharp. He did what he could and did not create an excuse otherwise. He could not run a marathon; however, he created multiple streams of exercise within his capabilities, and that created a big difference.

BEING FULFILLED

Who is going to tell you like it is? Who will allow you to become better than you are today? Even if you already exercise and don't smoke, look at the bigger picture. If things are not at the level you want them to be, then you have some work to do. Take what you just read about and expand it outside of this example of smoking and exercise. Ask: "What is the statement I create when I do _____?" You fill in the blank.

By not going out of your way each time you leave to kiss your spouse good-bye, what message does that send to him or her? By not putting down what you are doing when your children want to show you something they are proud of, what message does that send to them? How does this impact your relationships? By hitting the snooze button and choosing to sleep in and not exercise, what message does that send to your self-esteem? By consistently overeating when you are trying so hard to release weight, what message does that send you? How does this impact your results? How does this impact your business?

WHERE DO WE GROW FROM HERE?

This is the time where it is imperative you do some deep reflecting and some honest soul searching as to the concepts you read about in this book. This is your time to decide. Decide on where your main focus is most appropriate. Recognize the power of decision. If you break up the word decide, de–cide... *cide* is a Latin root meaning to kill off. Think of *pesticide* or *suicide*. A decision is to kill off all other possibilities.

Deciding on where your main focus is appropriate comes from your intuition. Honor how you feel and kill off any other possibility. Once you have done that, go back to the section where your focus is detailed and begin the process of the Seven Stages. Realize that the process can take years and is dynamic. Regularly reviewing the new model for fulfillment in Section One and the ten philosophies in Section Two are vital.

If you feel that you require assistance with your process of being fulfilled, take note of the resource section. There are many levels of resources, and the one that will assist you the most with this particular information is my nine-week *Being Fulfilled* Coaching Experience. This will unequivocally be your best resource for specifically applying this book's information in your world, with your focus. Congratulations on your dedication and commitment to yourself for completing this book. I look forward to hearing about your success and fulfillment.

The Beginning

While it may feel like the end to some of you, if you believe that you truly have the capacity to grow, it is only the beginning. In my office, just to the left of my desk is a photo a good friend gave me. On it is a quote by Albert Einstein:

"The *main* thing is to keep the *main* thing the *main* thing."

Cheers to you keeping your main thing your main thing and... *Being Fulfilled!*

ABOUT THE AUTHOR

Jeffrey St.Laurent is the founder of True You, Inc. Seminars and Coaching. He is an internationally recognized speaker, author, fitness trainer and business success coach. Jeff specializes in assisting success-minded business entrepreneurs increase profits and productivity by focusing on their number one asset: their mind and body. He calls this the Mind–Body–Prosperity Connection. Work harder on yourself than you do on your business, and you will experience dramatic results!

Once a shy, overweight, retiring young man, he was transformed through fitness and its power on the mind, body, and spirit. Recognizing the difference it made in his own life, he wanted to find a way to assist others in discovering their own unique formula for living a purposeful and passionate life.

He began as a personal trainer and lifestyle and weight management consultant. In time he added group fitness to the mix as an instructor and national trainer and presenter, traveling throughout North America giving seminars and providing education, motivation, all the while improving his teaching and coaching skills. His experience in the industry has allowed him such opportunities as taking his training business to the Nike World headquarters in Oregon.

Through his speaking and coaching, his passion for assisting people has turned into a fierce desire to EMPOWER people. As a success coach, Jeff will pull you away from your circumstances of life and allow you to take an authentic look at your health. Not simply the health of your body, but of your mind, spirit and relationships as well. Knowing that the real formula for change must come from within, Jeff will have you look inside your heart to create the types of changes that are sustained through your own strengths and insights.

Jeff has been featured on over seven educational fitness DVD's distributed around the world. He maintains a steady schedule of personal coaching clients and delivers keynotes and seminars for major companies such as State Farm. He is first and foremost an adoring husband and proud father. He loves playing with his yellow lab, Cosmo and cycling outdoors on both road and mountain.

toll free **866.544.4131**
www. T RUE Y OU N OW .COM

RESOURCES

The following pages contain some personal resources that will assist you with not only the implementation of the material presented in this book, but also your overall results in life. That being said, before I share what specifically I have to offer you, I want to contribute an outside resource that I personally recommend with the highest confidence and trust: my personal mentor and coach, Jeffrey Combs, the president and CEO of Golden Mastermind Seminars, Inc.

Jeffrey and his wife Erica are not only my publishers, but they have also assisted me and have contributed greatly to my personal and business success. I have personally coached and mentored with Jeffrey for over forty hours and have attended their signature workshop *Breakthroughs to Success* many times.

Breakthroughs is a two and a half day retreat for personal growth. Over these days, Jeffrey and Erica create a relaxed environment that is conducive to opening up and breaking through any limitations in your life. As a professional speaker and coach who has attended many seminars and workshops around the country for over a decade, I can honestly say that what Jeffrey and Erica teach has assisted me the most in producing tangible, real results. As an entrepreneur, that would be called a paycheck; in my life that would be called fulfillment!

To take advantage of what Jeffrey and Erica have to offer at Golden Mastermind Seminars, visit their website or call them toll free.

toll free 800.595.6632
WWW.GOLDENMASTERMIND.COM

COACHING | SEMINARS

TRUE YOU

Achieve amazing results in your life, right now!

BEING FULFILLED 9 WEEK COACHING EXPERIENCE

Imagine what it will feel like **Being Fulfilled** in all areas of your life!

What **value** do you place on experiencing sustained and unlimited wealth?

If you are **serious** about your results, **who will assist** you along your journey?

Jeffrey St.Laurent would like to have the opportunity to be your personal coach and assist you through the powerful stages and steps in this book. In your 9-Week personal coaching experience with Jeff, you will not only benefit from his expertise as one of the top health & fitness and mind-body experts in the country, but more importantly you will receive extreme value from his intimate understanding of the material in this book… and how to specifically apply it to your unique life!

toll free **866.544.4131**
www. **T**RUE **Y**OU **N**OW .com

When you have decided you deserve fulfillment, abundance and prosperity in your life, contact Jeff directly at **866.544.4131** about investing in your own 9-Week coaching experience. Be sure to mention the B*eing Fulfilled* coaching experience for a special package!

> *Note: In order to participate in this program you must have read this entire book.*

toll free 866.544.4131
www. TRUE YOU NOW .com

BEING FULFILLED   SEMINAR EXPERIENCE

*Can you even fathom the connection, energy and synergy your team will create by **Being Fulfilled** together?*

__Imagine__ the amazing results your team will produce when they are completely fulfilled in their lives… in and out of work!

__Who will you bring__ into your next meeting that will deliver energy and the results you are seeking?

Jeffrey St.Laurent would like to have the opportunity to be the keynote speaker at your next event to share and specifically implement the ideas and concepts in this book to your unique team or business. Jeff is one of the few speakers out there who does not come to your event with a "canned" speech. With Jeff, you will not get a beige power point, behind the podium type of speech. You will witness a dynamic, easy to listen and results orientated speaker.

toll free 866.544.4131
www.TRUEYOUNOW.com

He does in the moment speaking which truly creates a "live", one of a kind event! He uses his extensive coaching skills to enhance the learning and listens to the crowd to provide a seminar truly tailored to the people in attendance. Part of this special seminar experience includes meeting with Jeff individually over the phone before the event to discuss what is most appropriate for the specific objective and theme of your event.

> *For more details about the **Being Fulfilled** seminar experience, contact Jeff through his website or Toll Free number below.*

toll free 866.544.4131
www.TrueYouNow.com

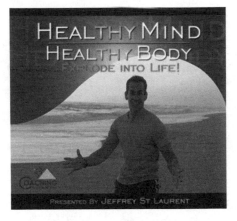

"I am slowly going through your most excellent CD series. Wow! Your testimony is very powerful and you have said some key things that have stuck with me...both personally and also for others benefit. I'm sure you are going to touch many people's lives by sharing this wisdom with others. I love every time I look at the cover and see your bright face!"

-**Gail,** Washington

"I finished listening to your CD series. Boy am I happy I purchased them! I already want to listen to Disc 7 again about reducing my Stress especially around work, I love it. I am still feeling thankful for the progress I have made since I started listening and have received some great feedback from my own children, my students, and their parents that I have made a difference in their lives."

- **Sharon,** Pennsylvania

Imagine what would be different in your life and how it would feel being able to write a testimonial like those! Visit our website below and listen to sample audio clips, learn disc by disc content and purchase!

www.TRUEYOUNOW.com

SHARE
BEING
FULFILLED
WITH YOUR TEAM

*Order a supply of **Being Fulfilled** to sell on your own or to give as gifts to friends, associates and relatives.*

If you are the owner of a business and are planning for rapid growth in the next few years, buy a copy of this book for *everyone* on your team. The momentum created by implementing these philosophies and stages *together*, will ensure that you reach your vision much sooner than ever anticipated!

Pricing already *includes* USPS 2-Day Priority shipping anywhere in the US!

1 Book	$25
5 Books	$94
10 Books	$159
15 Books	$205
20 Books	$234

Want a different quantity? Call for special pricing!

toll free **866.544.4131**
www.**BEINGFULFILLED**.NET

NOTES

_____

_____

_____

_____

_____

_____

_____

_____

_____

_____

_____

_____

_____

_____

_____

_____

NOTES

NOTES